Sickness in Health: Bullying in Nursing and other Health Professions

Brenda Happell

Sickness in Health: Bullying in Nursing and other Health Professions

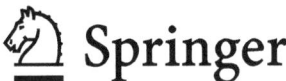 Springer

Brenda Happell
Happell Consulting
Merrijig, VIC, Australia

Faculty of Health
Southern Cross University
Bilinga, QLD, Australia
e-mail: brenda@happellconsulting.com.au

ISBN 978-3-031-49335-5   ISBN 978-3-031-49336-2   (eBook)
https://doi.org/10.1007/978-3-031-49336-2

This Springer imprint is published by the registered company Springer Nature Switzerland AG
The registered company address is: Gewerbestrasse 11, 6330 Cham, Switzerland

Paper in this product is recyclable

I dedicate this book to the 12 champions who shared some of the most distressing experiences of their lives and allowed me to tell their stories. To them and every health professional who has been bullied, this book is for you.

Preface

You've done something for all of us no one else would. You've treated us with compassion, support, and humanity. I am endlessly grateful (Alex).

The health professions are charged with responsibility for positively impacting the health and well-being of the communities they serve. It is, therefore, surprising to many that they experience some of the highest rates of bullying of all occupations. Even more concerning, most of the bullies are other health professionals who should be motivated by the desire to do good for others. I have witnessed bullying. I have experienced it far too often. It is not okay, and it needs to change. In what seems an insurmountable problem, it is my hope that this book will go some way to raising awareness about bullying and its impact. I hope this book will let those who are being bullied or who have been that they are not alone and that they are not responsible for what is happening to them. Bullying is not just a distasteful experience, it can be life changing, even life-ending. Targets of bullying need a voice. We need to show the people behind the statistics. I hope this book gives voice to people who have been bullied and raises awareness in bystanders. This is a book for all health professionals who seek a positive work environment where they can use their skills and knowledge to contribute to the health and well-being of their communities.

Merrijig, VIC, Australia   Brenda Happell
Bilinga, QLD, Australia

Acknowledgements

It sounds cliche to say so many people have contributed, directly or indirectly, to making this book a reality. I start by acknowledging Catherine, Judy, and Jennelle, managers, leaders, and mentors who believed in me and provided opportunities and support. You may never know how much you inspired me, and I am forever grateful.

My thanks to the people I worked with who were collegial, supportive, and shared my passion to make a positive difference to the world. I know how difficult it can be to shine in the face of toxicity. I can't name you all and I hope you know who you are.

Thanks to those who supported me during some tough times. You may not have realised that your small acts of kindness made such a difference. I did.

Sincere thanks to Brett for encouraging me to continue when I almost gave up. Trish, Aine, Patrick, Lynn, Clive, and John, thanks for taking the time to read the book and provide honest, supportive, and encouraging feedback. A special acknowledgement to John who helped me so much with writing style (as if supporting me during dark times wasn't enough). Thanks so much to Rasa for her assistance in finding a publisher.

I could never give enough thanks and praise to the 12 champions who offered me a window into their experiences and so willingly shared their stories of bullying and how it changed their lives. Thanks also for taking the time to read the book and provide suggestions and encouragement. Without you, this book would not have been possible.

Finally, to my family, especially my partner Steve and son Shannon, my greatest supporters, without whom I often wonder how I would have survived.

To anyone I have forgotten, my apologies and thank you.

Contents

About the Author

Brenda Happell grew up in the south-eastern suburbs of Melbourne with her parents and three siblings. Her answer to the question "What do you want to be when you grow up?" was "Author" without hesitation. She attended the local primary and secondary schools before commencing an Arts degree at La Trobe University in 1976. Over the next 20 years, she completed her Bachelor of Arts with Honours, a Diploma in Education, Certificates in general and psychiatric nursing, a Bachelor of Education, Masters in Education, and Doctor of Philosophy. She worked as a general nurse and secondary school teacher before finding her passion in mental health nursing. In 1990, Brenda began her academic career at Victoria College Burwood (later Deakin University). During her full-time academic career, Brenda worked at the University of Melbourne, Central Queensland University, and at the University of Canberra. She held many leadership positions, including the inaugural Director of the Centre for Psychiatric Nursing Research and Practice, Director of the Institute for Health and Social Science Research and Executive Director, Synergy: Nursing and Midwifery Research Centre. Brenda's academic career provided the opportunity to fulfil her ambition as an author, having written more than 500 journal articles, four books, and nine book chapters. She has received several awards including the Victorian Mental Illness Awareness Council, Lifetime Ally Award, and the Mental Health Services Award for Exceptional Achievement for Mental Health. Brenda retired from full-time work in 2018. She currently works part time as Professor of Mental Health, Southern Cross University and casually as a Senior Research Fellow at the University College Cork. She has also established her own business Happell Consulting. She manages her jobs and business remotely while living in her country retreat in Merrijig, Victoria. Brenda lives with her partner Steve. She enjoys travelling, writing, reading, spending time with her adult son Shannon and watching her football team, Carlton.

Introduction

After all these years, I can still see Andrew's face. He was a nursing student, a young man in his 20s, only months away from finishing his degree. His whole life was ahead of him. The news that he had taken his own life was devastating to all who knew him. I felt so much sadness for him and his family. A few days after his death, I was summoned to my boss's office. I was expecting some kind words and perhaps an offer of counselling. I sat directly opposite her. She was glaring at me. "How responsible do you feel for Andrew's death?" I will never forget these words. The tone of her voice made it clear this was not a question. It was an accusation. I went cold, numb. I had barely processed the news of his death, yet here I am, sitting across from an angry woman being blamed for it. "I don't feel responsible at all, but I have the impression you think I am". It was the best I could come up with at the time. My voice was shaking. I was shaking. She told me I was responsible because I had kept information from her, which had likely contributed to Andrew's decision to end his life. She would not accept my honest reassurance that I was not privy to the information I had supposedly withheld. All the devastation and sadness we felt about his death was now in my throat, choking me: was I responsible? Was my boss right? Could I have done something to change the outcome? Of course, we realised that none of us had anything to do with Andrew's tragic death. Had we seen it coming, as trained mental health professionals, we would have done everything possible to stop it. Why would my boss behave in this way? I don't know. I can say that she wasn't the first bully I had encountered in my career, like most, she had the knack of twisting whatever was at hand to denigrate and humiliate her colleagues at will. Through this book, I tell my story and those of 12 individuals who often endured horrendous abuse from so-called colleagues. These stories need to be told. It is time to expose what bullies always want: to keep their sneaky toxicity secret.

I did not recognise my boss's accusation as bullying. Our relationship deteriorated, and I was blocked from opportunities to advance my career. The thought of making a complaint never crossed my mind. I did my best to work around my boss and adjust to her lack of support. With the gift of hindsight, I see it for what it was,

© The Author(s), under exclusive license to Springer Nature
Switzerland AG 2024
B. Happell, *Sickness in Health: Bullying in Nursing and other Health
Professions*, https://doi.org/10.1007/978-3-031-49336-2_1

the actions of a bully. How did I not see it at the time? I still ask myself. I was a mental health nurse and a secondary school teacher, well-educated and informed about mental health issues. I was strong and resilient, yet I did not see it. Unfortunately, this bullying episode was not my last, far from it. I have seen and experienced the worst bullying by health professionals who should be motivated to provide the best possible health care to the community. They should be compassionate and caring, yet they are capable of such cruel and destructive behaviour.

I decided to write this book when I realised I was a victim of workplace bullying. I can't recall when I first heard the term. Bullying was what happened in schoolyards. Bullies would threaten or hit other kids, steal their lunch money, or humiliate them. Bullying was obvious. Everyone knew who the bullies were. They were the kids who seemed to relish making peoples' lives miserable. I was aware of bad behaviour in the workplace. I had seen and experienced it, yet I didn't think of it as bullying.

It was about a year before I retired. I was overwhelmed by the toxicity surrounding me. I felt trapped, and nothing I did seemed to work. I'd had a glass of wine or two and wondered why this was happening to me. So, I googled "am I being bullied?" I found a questionnaire from a psychology organisation. I'm not sure how reputable it was, but I decided to give it a go. Many questions were about being yelled at and subjected to rumours and threats. That hadn't been my experience. So, I was surprised to see the "results" that I was being overtly and consistently bullied. Then, it hit me! Wow, I have been bullied, and this has been happening for years. Strangely, there was relief that there was a name for what I had experienced. Even now, I can't believe it took that long to realise that what was happening to me was not just a few unfortunate and unrelated events. I now knew that I didn't cause it and it was not my fault. I have since discovered that not recognising the more subtle forms of bullying is not unique to me. The image of the schoolyard bully remains influential.

I spent considerable time reflecting on what I had previously considered unpleasant working environments. I realised that being excluded, ignored, micromanaged, belittled, undermined, and constantly facing changing goalposts and unreasonable work demands were all examples of workplace bullying. Indeed, these more subtle forms were more powerful because they were not easy to recognise and address. Sadly, in my profession of mental health nursing, bullying is rife. I reflected on the many occasions I was not given the information I needed to do my job. Resources promised to me were taken, often without discussion or explanation. The lack of support, not being told things I needed to know, and being excluded, time and time again. There was little doubt I had been bullied.

It came to the point that enough was enough, and I decided to retire. It was not the time or the way I wanted my career to end, but the long-term mental health impacts of persistent bullying caught up with me. I clearly remember my last official workday. I felt both enormous relief and a huge letdown. Finally, I was free. I would wake up the following Monday knowing I didn't have to ever subject myself to that all-consuming toxic environment again. It was time to reclaim myself and begin the process of healing. Yet, there was such sadness. The thought that I could have achieved so much more was never far from my mind in the following weeks. Sure, some of that is being a chronic overachiever and meeting my self-imposed goals, meaning I should set higher ones. But it was more than that. I felt an overwhelming sadness that bullying and toxicity had set up so many barriers. I spent so much time working around roadblocks, time I could have spent doing a better job and achieving more. I was frustrated by so many "colleagues". The very people who should be working with me so often worked against me. I was bewildered and shattered by the pervasive and unnecessary competitiveness I encountered and how often personality issues destroyed professional relationships. I didn't need people to like me. I just wanted to work with people using our mutual strengths to serve the organisation and the profession more broadly. I worked with many people who, had I discovered a miraculous cure for mental distress, would have dismissed it as unimportant, tried to discredit me, or at the very least refused to acknowledge the achievement. Whatever faults and failings I might have had, I was passionate about mental health nursing. I worked extremely hard, and I was successful. I have never been a back slapper or one of the girls, and I had no intention or desire to do so. All those traits no doubt went against me. I learned it's not what you do; it's who likes you.

Retirement gave me time to consider how bullying and toxicity were a part of my life for almost 30 years. Unfortunately, in all four of my full-time academic appointments, I experienced it at some point. I do not regret my career. It was wonderful. I had the opportunity to work with and for some brilliant and supportive people. They showed me what collegiality and leadership meant. That fairness and respect could prevail even in the cesspool many universities had become. They gave me hope.

I learned a lot about managers. Regrettably, I found many to be competitive, deceptive, and duplicitous. Some managers were the reason I left jobs. But, by reflecting through the lens of bullying, I realised I was not just unlucky. Some managers were threatened by successful team members, even though nurturing them would enhance their team's success. They could bask in that glory, knowing they had contributed to the environment that made it possible.

While my bullying experiences were hurtful, draining, and distracting, they also held a degree of fascination for me. I often found myself thinking—why are you doing this? What need in you does this behaviour meet? I was bemused and even flabbergasted that health professionals could be devoid of human caring and effective communication with colleagues. The skills that should have been the very core of their clinical practice were missing in action. What did they think when they created or maintained a toxic environment or bullied their colleagues? Did they ever reflect on their behaviour and question whether they had gone too far, even a little? Did they wonder if they had used their voice instead of their power, could the result have meant less distress and better outcomes for all? Did they ever consider how their actions affected the broader health service, profession, or university? Did the health and well-being of the people they bullied ever enter their minds? Did they believe their actions were justified or even the target's fault? Were they just sad, unfulfilled people who projected their unhappiness on others, particularly those more successful than themselves? Did they feel so threatened in their jobs that they needed to protect themselves? Ultimately, I wonder if these people considered

themselves to be bullies. Did they realise the environment they created or perpetu-
ated was toxic? Or was it just part of a pervasive culture that has surrounded them
in health, particularly in senior positions they have held? Have they become blind?

Amidst these episodes of bullying and toxicity, I continued, and my career was
successful. I always included colleagues in my activities, sometimes well above
what their contribution warranted. I believe I was an excellent mentor to students
and colleagues. Interestingly, many of the colleagues I did the most for were those
who later bullied me. I learnt to harden my shell, which was easier knowing that
these churlish and inaccurate assertions said much more about the people making
them than they did about me. What did hurt was managers who, for whatever reason, did not like me from the outset or turned from supporter to antagonist with no
apparent reason and no discussion. I honestly thought that health professionals
would have the skills and the desire to work things out. Maybe I was incredibly
naïve to believe they would be motivated by the greater good.

For the most part, I have loved my jobs. I loved the work, the variety, and the
autonomy. The decision to leave was always hard and meant saying goodbye to
much that was satisfying. —The saying—"people don't leave jobs, they leave managers"—could not have been truer for me. I could not endure being stifled, particularly when this stood in the way of doing good work. I had to get out.

To help me understand my situation, I did more reading and thinking about
workplace bullying. I knew it wasn't just me. I saw what had happened to colleagues and actively advocated for some. Realising the unrelenting effects of bullying and toxicity left me feeling I needed to do something. A story needed to be told.
It would have been easy to review the literature and come up with figures about the
rates of bullying within the health professions. I could have found media coverage
that described the toxic working conditions many health professionals endure. As a
researcher of 30 years, it might have been the obvious way to go. I didn't consider
it for long. Existing research describes the extent of bullying and, to some degree,
its consequences. The research tells us clearly that bullying is rife in health care.
Toxic workplaces are common, and bullying is now firmly part of the culture in
many organisations. I didn't want to do more of the same. I didn't want to write
papers that followed the formulaic structure with the necessary dissection of people's experiences into neat themes and sub-themes. I am not criticising the process,
which was essential to my work for many years. I wanted this book to be different.

I wanted to talk to people with bullying experiences, to be a conduit for them to
tell their stories. I wanted to present the human side. To show what it feels like when
constant bullying prevents you from doing the job you want to do, caring for people,
looking after students, and contributing to quality health services. I aspired to give
voice to their stories of how the traumatic effects of bullying didn't end when they
went home. I wanted to show the pervasive impact of bullying and toxicity on their
lives, the lives of the very people with responsibility for the health and well-being
of others. I wanted to tell these stories because they need to be told.

I can almost picture the looks on the faces of some people who have positioned
themselves as my adversaries at the thought of me writing a book about bullying. I
was accused of being a bully, twice to my face. Both times I was asking people to

be accountable. Interestingly, one was a person I consider one of the nastiest bullies I have ever encountered. The other was experiencing major life upheavals. If I had made a formal complaint, I could have easily refuted her accusations with extensive documentary evidence. I did not. I did not feel that would have been useful to either of us at the time.

So how am I so sure I'm not a bully? I expect many bullies would be shocked to be seen in that light. I wanted to be sure I was not one of those people and was not projecting toxic behaviour onto others. Reassuring myself meant going beyond understanding what bullying is to understand what it is not. Reasonable management action is not workplace bullying. While there is a fine line between reasonable and unreasonable, managers have a right to expect the people they supervise to do the job they are employed to do. They also have the right to take appropriate action where this does not occur. So long as the action is supportive and respectful, this is not bullying. What is essential to understand is that having different opinions, asking questions, and being assertive are not bullying behaviours. I am assertive, speak my mind, and communicate my views with confidence and vigour. I am polite and respect the opinions of others. People tell me I am persuasive. I consider that a compliment, whether intended or otherwise. I expect and welcome the same characteristics in others. I value honesty and am very comfortable with people disagreeing, countering my arguments, and presenting new evidence. I prefer someone tell me they dislike or find me difficult than smile to my face, hatchet me behind my back, ignore me, or treat me disrespectfully. Sure, I can be wrong, and others can outrank me. That's life, and I accept it. I don't accept being bullied or accused of bullying because of it. I could counter any accusation of bullying. The bullying I experienced could not be explained this way. I would welcome the opportunity to talk openly and honestly with those who have bullied me. I won't hold my breath.

I hope this book will emphasise the human experience of bullying and toxicity and give a voice to the people behind the statistics. Will it make a difference to the bullies? Probably not. What I do hope is that it gets people thinking and talking. I hope that targets of these toxic behaviours who, like me, have considered themselves unlucky or even responsible realise they are being bullied. I hope they see that what is happening to them is not okay and that they have a right to feel physically and emotionally safe at work.

Not all health professionals are bullies, and not all health environments are toxic. Those who work within unhealthy environments often desire change. I hope these people are sufficiently motivated to take action to create a more positive and constructive environment. At the very least, I want to contribute to the conversations about workplace bullying, to the understanding that people have a right to be treated respectfully at work. Enough is enough. The time to change toxic cultures is now.

1.1   The Champions

With great pleasure and a sense of privilege, I introduce you to the 12 people who generously shared their workplace bullying experiences with me. I call them champions. Champions are people who strongly support or defend a cause. Sharing their experiences of bullying and toxicity in health care and its impact on their lives makes them champions in my mind.

Finding people willing to tell their stories was more difficult than anticipated. I searched Facebook for pages and groups dealing with workplace bullying and harassment and joined several. I set up a Facebook page and group: bullying and toxicity in the health professions, and a Twitter account, @bullyhealth, as none of the existing social media accounts explicitly related to health professions. I later set up a LinkedIn page. I posted on my own and other Facebook pages and groups, asking people to contact me if they were willing to share their stories. The response was slow. Some people contacted me through social media, and one became the first champion. I chatted with others on social media for a while, and ultimately, they decided not to be involved. One person didn't feel well enough. Another wanted to tell her story but was worried colleagues would recognise her. Others said they would contact me when they were ready and did not make further contact.

I may have given up if not for Rory. Perhaps people were not interested. Maybe they were too distressed to share painful experiences or were concerned their story would be recognised and management would punish them. They may not have trusted me—all perfectly understandable. Rory was so generous with her time; she sent me a comprehensive written summary of her situation and additional documentation. Her story was poignant and strongly impacted her work and personal life. She motivated me to continue this work.

Slowly people began to join my Facebook group, retweet my tweets, and comment on my postings on other pages. I started sending private messages to people who commented, telling them more about what I was doing and asking if they would like to talk to me. Gradually people said yes. Some champions passed my details on to colleagues, and over the following months, I had taped conversations with 12 champions. I had at least two and up to four follow-up conversations with each, some lasting for hours. Some champions sent notes and other documents. They were amazingly generous and trusting, and I thank them sincerely. It was an honour to be entrusted with their stories.

The champions related their stories in vivid detail, many heartbreaking to hear. I found myself feeling guilty that I dared consider myself badly treated. I shouldn't complain. I had to remind myself that this was not a competition. Everyone has a right to go to work, be treated with respect, feel safe, and have every opportunity to do a good job. I, too, had been bullied, and no amount of bullying is acceptable.

Now to the champions themselves. When telling stories, it is customary to introduce people using a pseudonym and describe their discipline background, career summary, length of experience, and more personal details such as gender and age. Revealing these details would be risky. Some champions still work in or have strong connections with the health industry. Some are still employed by the toxic organisation, while others have ongoing complaint processes. Confidentiality is essential for them. With their permission, I am using pseudonyms. I have chosen unisex names, and gender is not specified unless by the champion. I use the pronouns she/her for all champions other than Terry, who identifies as male in his story. At Taylor's request, I am using the non-gendered language them/they/their for the people she describes in her story. Despite best efforts, someone reading this book may recognise a story and think wow, that is Chris. They may be right. They might also be thinking of someone who has unfortunately had experiences similar to Chris's. Despite the uniqueness of everyone's experience, sadly, there are many common ways bullying impacts people. Every champion had something in their story that I'd observed or experienced at some point. Many health professionals will feel the same. The champions have reviewed the book and are comfortable with the final version.

The champions were all living in Australia at the time of our conversations. They had been bullied at least once in this country. They were located across Australia; some had worked in more than one state or territory. The champions worked in different roles, including clinical practice, management, and academia. Most had 20 or more years of experience with career lengths from around five years to 40. I will briefly introduce each champion and their discipline background and bullying experiences.

Alex worked as an emergency medical dispatcher with ambulance services. She was assaulted by a colleague soon after commencing her training. After reporting the assault, a tirade of persistent and intrusive bullying was unleashed from all levels of the organisation. Alex was on WorkCover for several years until her legal action against the organisation was finally settled.

Andy is a registered nurse. Her story includes two significant incidents of persistent bullying by managers. The first time Andy's honesty and openness appeared to be the trigger. The second came from a misunderstanding that seemed to have labelled Andy a troublemaker and a fair target.

Chris is a mental health nurse. She was a new graduate the first time a registered nurse bullied her. She worked in a clinical role for the second time, and her positive relationship with her manager changed dramatically. Unfortunately, the bullying continued until she resigned. Chris was bullied for the third time by another boss. She was one of many singled out as a target in what had become a very toxic environment.

Jesse completed a degree in psychology before moving into public health. Her manager bullied her for the first time after they applied for the same position, and he was successful. After moving into the university sector, Jesse was bullied by her boss in two successive university appointments. She is now semi-retired.

Jordan is a registered nurse who spent most of her career in academic roles. Successive bosses, colleagues, and staff bullied her. Her roles often extended across departments and organisations, with several reporting lines and reliance on external funding, which made her situation more complicated. Therefore, Jordan found it hard to know where to start dealing with bullying. She was also actively engaged in her broader professional communities, where bullying extended further. She is now retired.

Lee has a background in psychology. She spent most of her career in mental health research, where she experienced bullying and witnessed it happening to colleagues. She moved into an education and training role with a boss who bullied staff, and Lee was a primary target.

Pat is a social worker. She had experienced bullying frequently. However, our conversations focused mainly on one example. She had worked at the organisation for many years. After returning from extended leave following surgery and a life-threatening illness, her new manager seemed to dislike her instantly, and the bullying began. Pat subsequently left and is working as a social worker in another role. She is enjoying the new position and not experiencing bullying.

Rory is a medical doctor. At the time of her bullying, she was in training to specialise in a specific field of medicine. Unfortunately, a personality clash with an influential staff member progressed to bullying at multiple levels. Once Rory made a formal complaint, the situation worsened, and she was forced out. She now works at another hospital and is finding the environment very positive. Rory's circumstances were particularly complicated because of multiple reporting lines relating to rotations in specific clinical areas, her education program, mentorship, and line management.

Sam is a mental health nurse. She has worked successfully in the same organisation for many years in clinical, professional development, and management roles. Sam has a mutually respectful relationship with her direct manager. She reports professionally to the senior nurse who has bullied her for some time.

Shannon is a mental health nurse. She was first bullied when her manager overheard a comment she made to a colleague. When management took formal action, Shannon found the environment so challenging that she took extended leave and ultimately resigned. The second time she was bullied by peers over an extended period. She recently resigned and now works in a new and very positive environment.

Taylor's background is as a peer worker. In these roles, she uses her lived experience of mental distress to support people accessing services for their mental health needs. Taylor has experienced intense and sustained bullying throughout her career, both in the workplace and through her broader professional activities. She is now in a senior executive position in a designated lived experience role. Taylor's lived experience is valued and facilitates positive change. Despite her bullying experiences, she has continued to be successful in her career.

Terry is a mental health nurse. Most of his career has been in academic roles in his home country. Terry first experienced bullying as a nursing student. He moved to Australia a few years ago to take up a research position between a university, health service, and a not-for-profit organisation. The bullying was particularly challenging because of multiple reporting lines and complex systems. Terry now works for another Australian university and has found the environment more positive.

After the first couple of drafts of this book, I chose to tell my own story. I related to many of the champions' experiences, and it seemed wrong to hide behind them. I became braver because of them and overcame my reluctance to speak of what happened to me, to reveal so much that is personal and was still profoundly hurtful. It is obvious who I am, so I have been selective, sharing what I feel comfortable with and avoiding shedding a negative light on specific people and organisations. I have also been careful not to dominate and constantly remind myself that the focus is on conveying the stories of others.

The experiences presented by the champions are taken at face value, as their experiences and how they were affected. Readers will likely have their own views about if or how these experiences would pass a legal or reasonable person test as bullying. I have not judged or analysed them. Instead, they represent the traumatic events these 12 people considered as bullying.

It is now time to hear from the champions themselves. I use their words as close to word for word without potentially identifying them. The point of the book is to give voice to their experiences, and there is no one better to tell a story than those who have lived it.

A final word before we begin. It is often said, "there are two sides to every story". Indeed, there are multiple sides. While I would have dearly loved to hear these experiences through the eyes of the people identified as bullies, this was not possible or practical. I did amuse myself with the thought of contacting people I believed bullied me. If they were willing to engage with me, they would likely not see themselves as bullies and much less want to talk about how their tactics and actions affected me. There is no suggestion that this book presents the absolute truth. There is no need to do so. These words convey how people feel about bullying and working in toxic workplaces. They are true for them. I hope this book reflects that.

Becoming a Health Professional

2

I wanted to do something productive and meaningful for society (Rory).

Why do people become health professionals? The reasons are no doubt as complex and varied as the people themselves. In researching this book, I was surprised so little has been written about this. Therefore, my thoughts and opinions are mainly anecdotal, from my career and working with clinicians, students, and researchers from nursing and other health disciplines. However, research tells us that people consider health professions among the most trustworthy. While this alone might not explain decisions, it may be an influence. Opportunities to work with people and contribute to positive change are strong drawcards. Some people, having experienced illness or adversity themselves or through supporting a family member, wanted to be just like the professionals that helped on their journey. For others, a stable career, at least reasonably well paid, offering secure employment and opportunities for working holidays were very appealing. Finally, some wanted to be a health professional from childhood, while others decided later in life.

I started my conversations with the champions by asking about their decision to become a health professional. It was an opportunity to get to know them and provide some background to understand their experiences of bullying and toxicity. Some conversations led to their reasons for choosing the speciality or setting where they now worked. We also talked about any images they had of the profession and working environment before they commenced. I hope you will get to know them better through these stories as I did.

2.1 Motivations

With no expectations whatsoever, I did psychology, got a high distinction, and topped the honours year. That's how by pure accident (Jesse).

© The Author(s), under exclusive license to Springer Nature Switzerland AG 2024
B. Happell, *Sickness in Health: Bullying in Nursing and other Health Professions*, https://doi.org/10.1007/978-3-031-49336-2_2

The champions came to their careers in health through different and varied paths. A career as a health professional was seen as "ticking all the boxes" for Rory and Lee although Rory was initially reluctant:

Rory: My dad's a doctor, and I spent my childhood saying I'm not going to be a doctor because of dad not being around much. I became very interested in science and loved biology, human physiology, and physical education. I ended up with this list of goals of a profession I wanted, essentially the description of medicine or allied health. I wanted to work with people. I wanted to do something productive and meaningful for society. I wanted to be stimulated and do something interesting, so it would always be medicine, physiotherapy, paramedics, or something in the field.

Lee: What attracted me was the opportunity to help people and the fact that it had a very strong scientific base. Many of the models we use in research have come from psychology. I like the art, the science, the flexibility, and there were so many parts to it.

Traumatic experiences and other life events seen or experienced attracted Pat, Sam, Lee, and Taylor towards a career in health. They saw it as a way to make a difference and contribute meaningfully:

Pat: I experienced the trauma of losing a baby. He was born early and died when he was two days old. The social worker was just lovely. She was so gentle and softly spoken and very caring. And I wanted to provide that support for a bereaved parent. I didn't want a bereaved parent to experience the feelings I had without support, so that spurred me to further study. I developed postnatal depression during my third pregnancy. My counsellor said: "You should do social work because you've got all these life skills, and you'd be really good at it". I thought, well, I've been out of school for a long time, and it's been a while since I've written an essay. I'll start small. I did a diploma in community services welfare. When I graduated, one of the ladies I went through the course with said, "You know what? We can do social work. We'll get about 18 months' recognition of prior learning". That's how I became a social worker.

Sam: A couple of my friends passed away when I was about 14 or 15. A couple by drug overdoses and one by their own hand. And it made you think, could you use these experiences to make a difference in people's lives? People often talk about mental illness coming from a poor upbringing and dysfunctional families. I believe those things sometimes give you strengths you wouldn't have had without those early challenges. I come from what may be described as a dysfunctional family. So some of the strengths I developed are probably because of that.

Lee: I've known some friends of my older sister. When I was young, one guy became a bit psychotic. It all seemed very crude in the sense that there was nothing done, no therapies, and not much treatment.

Taylor: I started my career as a peer worker after the death of my brother, who had the same diagnosis as me. I had been told that it runs in the family. So, I was concerned that my girls might get bipolar. I wanted to show them there was a way of living well and doing something meaningful and purposeful rather than not living well and dying with it. I didn't know that such a thing as a peer worker existed until I met a peer leader. I told them the psychiatrist told me I would never work and would never be a valuable member of society. And they, in a very gentle, loving way, challenged me. They said "I've got that same diagnosis, and I work, and I own my own home and car. So, why can't you do that?" And that really ignited my recovery, as well as my desire to work in that field. It was like a rebirth and a fierce calling all at once.

My own motivations to become a nurse were far from altruistic. Ironically, I wanted to be an author. My mother, in her infinite wisdom, told me that was very nice, but I would need a proper job (subtext: something I would make money from), and I fixed on journalism. After witnessing the brutal side of journalism, I fell out of love with that idea. I went to university to do an arts degree with only vague and transient ideas about what I wanted to do. I discovered, among other things, that I really loved studying and would have happily continued as a student forever if it weren't for that little thing about making a living. So, influenced by a love of studying and a desire to one-day travel the world, I decided to train as a nurse. I would still be paid, and I was setting myself up for a career where I was confident of finding work anywhere in the world. Nursing started as a means to facilitate my career, and in the end, it became my career.

Like me, Andy, Terry, and Jordan had been opportunistic, either because their first choice was not attainable or as a means to achieve other life goals.

Andy: When I started nursing, I had no idea what I wanted to do. I got into university to study genetics but financially couldn't do that. My sister was a nurse, and I chatted with her about it. I had always been sympathetic. So, I fell into it as a second choice. I thought nursing would be a great job, a job that would be for life. Nurses were well-respected and had the opportunity to learn and travel. This would be good for me. I could do all those things.

Terry: When I was young, I was in a car crash and had mild PTSD [Post Traumatic Stress Disorder]. After that, my school scores were completely rubbish, so I ended up in nursing, where all my mates became lawyers and doctors. So, everything got turned upside down because of that event.

Jordan: To be honest, I was looking for something to do. A friend told me he was starting nursing, and I thought, what a great idea. When I was at uni and living on campus, a student was an enrolled nurse. I was jealous of how she could work a few shifts here and there to pay the bills. So, I put in my application, and the rest is history.

Alex started work in ambulance services in a short-term administrative job and was encouraged by her manager to move into a healthcare-focused role:

> My manager encouraged me to apply as an Emergency Medical Dispatcher. He knew I had an interest, he knew it was something I wanted to do, and he encouraged it, so I did.

Surprisingly, Jesse found her lifelong career choice less attractive than she had expected. When looking for other options, she discovered her alternative path by accident:

> That's a very interesting story. I was doing a straight Science Degree. From the age of seven, I'd been going to be an Industrial Chemist. I got into second year of organic chemistry, and it was just the most boring thing on earth. I did not do well and had to pick up a subject. The choices were biology or psychology. I said to my older sister, "You've done both; which do you reckon?" And she said, "Oh, well, psychology's interesting". So, with no expectations whatsoever, I did psychology, got a high distinction, and topped the honours year. Maybe it just suited me. That's how by pure accident.

Sam's progression into a career in nursing was gradual and driven by working in health-related roles. Through these experiences, she became aware of human distress and a desire to contribute to people's health and well-being:

> I left school at 15 and worked in a pharmacy with a gentleman who had a significant bipolar disorder, undiagnosed for the first eight years. He would do bizarre things, like come into work naked with a fish on his head after drinking four litres of alcohol. It was an interesting time, and I wanted to understand what was behind it for him. I then worked in a doctor's surgery as a receptionist. I met this lady whose husband had died. He had done everything for her forever, so she was lost. She didn't know how to bank; she didn't know how to do anything. She came into the surgery one day and was extremely distressed and wanted to see the doctor, and there was no doctor there. As she left, she said, "I can't, I can't do this anymore". I was really worried about her. I rang the lady doctor and said I wanted to close the surgery and go and see if she was okay. She agreed and met me at the lady's place. She had attempted suicide. She felt there was nothing—she didn't know how to live. From there, I did my enrolled nursing in aged care. I developed a massive interest in mental health. We were busy ensuring that our people were clothed and bathed, their teeth were clean, and they were toileted whether they wanted to go or not. I wanted to do something different. I was fortunate to get a position in mental health. I always wanted to work in developmental psychiatry because I felt that if you could get in early, you could make a difference and change the trajectory of somebody's life.

Shannon had no idea what to do for a job, let alone a career. She was encouraged into nursing by a colleague who saw something in her she did not see herself:

> I finished Year 12, and I didn't get a job, and my mother said if you don't get a job, you will have to move out. So, she found me a job as a nursing assistant. I was a glorified tea lady, but I just loved it. And the nurse in charge decided to enrol me in this pilot program, the Bachelor of Applied Science in psychiatric nursing. And that's how I fell into it. It wasn't something I'd even known existed, to be honest.

Chris, having no thoughts about what she wanted to do after school, was persuaded by her mother to consider nursing:

> I fell into nursing accidentally. It was halfway through year 12, and you had to put in your preferences to go to uni, and I had no clue what I wanted to do. Mum said, "Look, I think you should just put down nursing because you love to help people, and you've got a caring nature, you want to travel, and that's a profession you'll be able to travel with". So reluctantly, I put nursing down, not thinking that was what I wanted to do. It wasn't until second year that I was glad I went the nursing route. It was my mother who knew me best.

2.2   Becoming a Specialist

> In second year, we completed our mental health placement. I had an amazing placement. And I just knew from that point on that, yep, yep, yep, I wanted to do mental health nursing (Chris).

My first job as a registered nurse quickly confirmed that general nursing was not for me. The thing I enjoyed most was the people contact. In a busy surgical ward, I didn't have much opportunity for that. I remember one day, at the end of the shift, I reflected that one "bed" I was allocated had three people that day. The first person was discharged soon after I came on shift, the second was admitted for day surgery and discharged shortly after, and the third was admitted before the day finished. I barely had time with any of them. I was confident I looked after their physical needs. Still, anything could have been happening emotionally, and I had no idea. It was too much like a sausage factory for me. Down the track, I got a job in a drug and alcohol service, and I loved it. It was a fantastic team and fulfilling work, just what I wanted. I realised my limitations, though, and I knew I had a lot to learn about communicating with people in distress. Psychiatric nursing, as it was then, was clear—a decision I have never regretted.

Chris and Terry made their decision to specialise in mental health nursing after a very positive clinical experience:

Chris: In second year, we completed our mental health placement. I had an amazing placement. And I just knew from that point on that, yep, yep, yep, I wanted to do mental health nursing. You had time to get to know and really understand people. At uni, I was learning all about person-centred care. In reality, in the general wards, I didn't get to focus on the patient because it was task orientated, and I had little time. Whereas mental health was never like that. The other thing I liked about mental health was that it seemed so collaborative. As a grad nurse, I can remember sitting in a clinical review for a patient, and the director of the clinical service turned to me and said, "What do you think? You've been working closely with this person". And me just sitting there thinking, "What, you actually care what I think?" The hierarchies did not feel the same in mental health compared to the general setting.

Mental health was not Terry's first choice. Instead, workplace conflict in his preferred area was the final push in that direction:

> Why mental health nursing? I enjoyed my work there, but I also enjoyed my final placement and thought I would continue in that kind of role. I returned to mental health nursing after a conflict with management in my final placement.

Jesse was motivated to pursue her career in public health because she was more interested in people than rats:

> I did apply for PhDs in psychology, but I hadn't done the work of getting myself ingratiated with someone, even though I was top of the year. My honours was in rats, and I went, oh my God, show me the people, where are they? I don't like chopping rats' heads off. I don't like any of this. So, population health sounded good because there were lots and lots of people.

2.3   Becoming an Academic

> What I was saying as a new graduate nurse is pretty much the same as I'm saying now. Because I've got a PhD, people listen to me. (Terry).

It was probably inevitable that I would become an academic. I loved university life since the day I started in 1976. I loved the freedom and the opportunity to write and think. I didn't immediately consider, "this is where I want to work", but it was always in my mind. During my nursing training, I was aware of the educators' teaching styles. It was like going straight back to high school with most of them, dull and monotonous. So, my positive and negative educational experiences led me to an academic career. I could teach, I could do research, and, oh yes, I could write! I could be an author, after all!

For other champions, transitioning from clinical practice into academia was an escape from the culture of the broader health system. It presented a welcome move for Terry from a toxic environment. It allowed him to be heard and respected instead of punished for his opinions:

> A pattern was starting to erupt. I ended up in conflict with the people I worked with because I found how patients were treated inhumane. Whenever I would object to that, I would be sanctioned heavily. That was one of my first experiences of really being sanctioned by a system that I found to be inhumane, but I was so sure that I had a valid point to bring forward. In my final year, I was allowed into the masters program. It came as a huge relief. Thinking back, what I was saying as a new graduate nurse is pretty much the same as I'm saying now. Because I've got a PhD, people listen to me. They say, "Oh, that's really good and interesting", but when I said it working as a grad nurse, I was making trouble.

Jesse sought refuge from a bully by taking a short-term contract at a university. The conditions were less favourable than the position she held. Still, it offered some respite from her negative working situation:

A friend at a university said, "Come and work for me. I've got a 10-month contract". So, I went on secondment. I actually had a drop in pay, a drop in level, because I just had to get out.

An academic career had been a long-term goal for Jordan, and nursing provided a convenient pathway:

I did an arts degree before nursing, a long time ago when universities were more like learning institutions and less like businesses than they are now. I loved the debates. We were encouraged to be critical and to think. My nursing training was in the old hospital-based system, and I did a lot of rote learning to pass the exams. It was boring. When nursing went to the universities, I thought this was my opportunity. I enjoyed the clinical work but loved the idea of teaching and research. It allowed me to do things differently and make a difference, so university was the obvious choice.

2.4   Image of Health Professionals

The social workers I worked with were very softly spoken and nurturing. I think for parents, it was like being wrapped in someone's arms and gently supported through their journey (Pat).

I certainly didn't go into nursing blindly. My mother had trained as a nurse in the 1940s, and I grew up with stories of the horrific conditions and rigid hierarchies she endured. She was working six 12-h shifts a week and studying on top. She talked about living in the nurses' home and being woken in the middle of the night if there was even the most minor task she had forgotten or, more likely, not had time to do. Not being a submissive person by nature, I worried about coping in such a strict environment. I expected it would have become a bit less extreme over the years. Still, I anticipated the worst. So much so that on my first day of nursing school in 30° heat, I wore pantyhose and sensible shoes, thinking we would have to change into our uniforms for class! The good thing about expecting the worst is a pleasant surprise. It was so much better than I had imagined. I did encounter some strict and unfriendly charge sisters. Some environments, like operating theatre, I had initially thought would interest me, were far too hierarchical. Still, the thought of bullying didn't cross my mind. Like me, Andy and Sam had little idea of what the professional and work environment would be:

Andy: I had no idea, really. My sister never really told me about anything in that respect, and I thought this would be hard work. But in terms of anything broader than that, I had no idea.

Sam: I didn't have any inkling other than just wanting to look after the patients. I didn't think, "This is going to be awful. This is going to be extreme".

Pat expected social workers would be like those who supported her through her grief and the incredible caring people she had worked with as a volunteer:

> I completed training to be a parent support person and a group leader in a voluntary organisation. The social workers I worked with were very softly spoken and nurturing. I think for parents, it was like being wrapped in someone's arms and gently supported through their journey.

Being Bullied

3

I don't think I even really knew to formulate that this was workplace bullying. I just knew that she was horrible, and I didn't want to work with her (Chris).

With increased attention to workplace bullying and its impact, it is essential to understand what this term means. The Australian Fair Work Commission identifies workplace bullying as occurring when: an individual or group of individuals repeatedly behaves unreasonably towards a worker or group of workers at work and the behaviour risks health and safety.

Bullying must be distinguished from reasonable management action, taken to ensure workers fulfil the requirements of their job, where appropriate policies and procedures are followed. While this is not always an easy distinction, it provides a useful starting point. The risk to health and safety is not confined to physical harm and includes matters financial, emotional, and sexual.

Increased attention to workplace bullying in the health professions has revealed alarmingly high rates. Health and community services are consistently identified as experiencing workplace bullying at one of Australia's highest levels of occupational groups. For example, in nursing, it is estimated that as many as 59% have witnessed bullying at work, with almost half being directly affected as targets. Twelve per cent of those reported experiencing bullying several times a week. In medicine, the reported rates are around 50%, with junior doctors likely to experience bullying more frequently. Managers and senior clinicians are the main perpetrators in both professions. I was unable to find Australian data for social work. However, international figures suggest rates of bullying between 22 and 59%. I was not able to find data for other professions.

While writing this book, bullying in ambulance services in Australia, particularly in Victoria and New South Wales, hit the media. The available data doesn't show the proportion of staff affected; however, it does show that bullying-related violence and assaults are increasing exponentially. Amidst a description of a hostile and toxic culture, many cases likely go unreported.

B. Happell, *Sickness in Health: Bullying in Nursing and other Health Professions*, https://doi.org/10.1007/978-3-031-49336-2_3

Employers, managers, or people who hold prominent positions of power over the target are common perpetrators of bullying. Bullying can also occur from peer to peer, commonly known as horizontal violence. It can involve individuals or groups (known as mobbing). More recently, upward bullying has been identified as when people bully their managers or others in positions of authority. Because of my experience and those of others, I am taking an expansive definition of workplace bullying, including broader professional and voluntary roles. These work-related, extra-curricular activities have yet to be widely considered sites for bullying, as I suspect they should be.

This chapter presents some broad experiences and types of bullying: as students or new graduates, downward, horizontal, upward, and mobbing, and bullying within broader professional and voluntary activities. The content of other chapters includes more specific details of the tactics bullies used, the impact of the toxic environment on the champions, and how they tried to deal with their experiences.

3.1   Experiences of Bullying

Following the light globe moment when I realised I was being bullied and not for the first time, I reflected on my career and the behaviours I had witnessed and experienced. I understood firsthand that bullying was rife in the health professions. The more I reflected and read, the more behaviours I recognised as bullying. I realised I had been bullied by managers and others in positions of power, peers, and people who worked for me. I had been bullied at work and in my broader professional circle. It wasn't just me—I had witnessed or heard about many colleagues being bullied. Talking with the champions further opened my eyes to bullying within the professions charged with creating a healthier community. Their experiences were widespread and occurred at different stages, from students to later periods in their careers. The bullying came from people in authority, peers, colleagues, and sometimes people working for them.

3.2   Bullied as Students and New Graduates

My clinical teacher was just horrendous ... very abrupt and rude. There were lots of coming home from shifts crying (Chris).

Students and new graduates are common targets of bullying, particularly in nursing and medicine. Research suggests at least 50% of nursing and 30% of medical students are bullied, most commonly during clinical placements. I have no recollection of being bullied as a student or in my clinical roles, either in general or in mental health. However, Terry experienced bullying for the first time as a student:

The ward was badly run. A lot of the people I was working with were new graduates, and they sucked me into the politics. I was invited to informal staff meetings where staff discussed what to do with their manager, who was hopeless. In time, someone told the ward manager what was going on, and the head nurse decided to make me an example and punished me. I just thought she was picking on the easy target because none of us were really meant to be at those meetings. Someone told her that I'd been there.

Chris was bullied for the first time during her graduate nurse year. Her clinical teacher, whose role it was to support her transition into the profession, singled her out for treatment very different to her peers:

> In my second rotation in my grad year, my clinical teacher was just horrendous. She was a bully. She spoke to me very differently from how she spoke to others, very abrupt and rude. I'd never experienced that before. It was really a very eye-opening experience. There were lots of coming home from shifts crying.

3.3   Downward Bullying

> I rang the manager and said I wanted to find out where I would be sitting when I return on Monday. And the words out of her mouth were, "You've got bigger problems than where you're going to be sitting" (Pat).

Bullying by managers, or others in positions of authority or influence, is identified as the most common form of workplace bullying. I have had so many managers during my career; sadly, only three stand out as exceptional. These managers showed faith in me, encouraged me to take opportunities, supported and helped me become more confident in my skills and talents, take risks and recognise my limitations and areas I needed to develop further. I am forever indebted to them. I am not suggesting we never experienced conflict. They made no bones about letting me know when I had stuffed up. I preferred it that way. What I saw was what I got, and once it was said, it was said, and we could move on. I have always been receptive to feedback. I have actively asked for it and learned a great deal from it.

There were two or three bosses who were not particularly supportive but did not cause me any real grief, and the remainder I now recognise as bullies. Interestingly, I'd have described some of them as supportive and approachable bosses when we first worked together until the tide turned. Although it took a long time for me to understand and recognise workplace bullying, I did learn the difference that management and leadership styles made to my job satisfaction, productivity, and well-being. I could see the negative impact of toxic management on me, other staff, and, more importantly, on the outcomes for the organisation itself.

Following my first experience of bullying, my career became one of cycles. I would have a great boss, be doing well, enjoying my work, and achieving great things, and then it would come crashing down around me. Along came a new boss who, for whatever reason, would not like me and would go out of their way to put blocks in my path, slow me down, and make everything about the job a long hard slog. I loved all my jobs at university, and I left every single one because of the bullying and toxicity.

My experience was far from unique. One or more bosses had bullied all champions. Jesse described her first experience when she and a colleague applied for the same position. He was successful, became her boss, and proceeded to bully her:

> I was employed as a middle manager by a health service, and I was really respected by my female boss. When she left, I applied for her job. Also, a male colleague applied. He'd just finished his PhD when I'd started mine, and he told me on one occasion that I was dangerous. I assume he was threatened by me. So it came to pass that he became my boss. And he just gave me an amazingly hard time. He really didn't want me there. He found me incredibly threatening.

When the bullying became overwhelming, Jesse sought refuge in an academic position where she was bullied again. Unfortunately, her new boss used Jesse's achievements for her own benefit:

> She used me up completely. And I let her, and I did it on the understanding that eventually good things would come to me, but I didn't ever get good things coming to me. We spent the next two to three years building a research program. She was the face of the program, and I was the one who did the background work. Everything in her name, right? When the program took off successfully, I was left behind.

After 10 years and helping to establish a very successful program, Jesse was told there was no further funding for the position. It was time to move on to a new role. Unfortunately, there was more bullying to come:

> She was a maddening boss, just maddening. One day, she's your best mate, and one day, she's your big boss and anything that happened on the day she was your best mate, that's not the way it is because she's your big boss. I could never tell where I was with her.

When Pat returned to work after a long illness and brain surgery, she decided to contact the new manager of her team to check in. The response was surprising and alarming to Pat:

> I rang the manager and said I wanted to find out where I would be sitting when I return on Monday. And the words out of her mouth were, "You've got bigger problems than where you're going to be sitting".

After many years of working long hours, with tight deadlines and high stress levels, Lee started a new job with reduced hours and a more manageable workload. All went well in the early stages until a change of management resulted in a toxic and bullying culture:

> When I first got there, it was Nirvana. We had a very nice boss. She was actually doing her PhD on mental health in the workplace. So, there was a vibe in the place. Anyway, the boss left. The new boss arrived and was nicey-nicey at first. Then things began to unravel. She started doing the classic bullying.

Some champions experienced bullying when trying to protect the rights of others. For example, the first time Shannon was bullied, she had warned a colleague to wear a jacket around a male staff member, hinting that he had a reputation for sexually inappropriate behaviour. Her manager, a good friend of the male staff member concerned, overheard the conversation and reported her to human resources:

> The next day there was a note from HR in my pigeonhole saying that a formal complaint had been put in about me. My manager had overheard me, and they were very good friends. I went to him and said, "Holy crap. I've got to see HR at 3 o'clock. Can you please be my independent third person?" And he said, "No. I was the one who put the complaint in". And he just gave it to me. He said, "It was totally inappropriate".

Relationship difficulties with managers were at the core of many bullying experiences. Andy had wanted to be upfront with her new boss. She wanted her to know she had not applied for the manager role and was not a competitor. This statement seemed to trigger the boss:

> I was the assistant manager, and the manager left. I didn't want that job, but I did that role until they appointed someone. They appointed a new centre manager, and oh my God, she was just incredible. So, I decided to make it quite clear from the outset that "I'm very happy that you're here. This isn't a job that I wanted. It's not a job that I applied for. I'm here to support you. I've been here for a long time". And she immediately said, "Well, since you're not interested in this job, even when I go on holidays, you can't do it", and it's just started from there. It just became extremely toxic.

A misunderstanding gave rise to Andy's second experience of bullying. She sought advice from the union about a long-standing workplace issue. Unfortunately, the matter was referred to her manager, and their previous close, professional relationship broke down:

> I rang the union to ask for advice about what I should do, not asking them to do anything. "Please call me and just tell me what I should do, how I should handle this because this has been going on for years". Unfortunately, the person didn't call me back. They rang the HR department. HR came over, and she got in trouble, and then she asked us who had rung the union, and I had to say it was me. I said, "Well, what happened was not my intention". From that moment onwards, that was it, very subtle but passive-aggressive bullying the whole time. I went from someone she would refer to as "my rock, my most dependable person that turns up all the time, that does the best job" to being the person that was put in whatever lab was the busiest for that day. Any time there was an opportunity to progress to a higher position, she would not accept my application.

3.4   Peer-to-Peer Bullying

> These women decided I was not wanted there and would do everything they could to … oust me from that building at any cost (Alex).

Bullying from peer-to-peer, commonly referred to as horizontal violence, involves an employee deliberately bullying a colleague of a similar position within the organisation. This form of bullying is increasingly recognised in health services, particularly nursing. Bullying is a major reason nurses consider leaving the profession and has far-reaching implications for health and well-being. It can be overt, involving physical, sexual, and verbal abuse or more subtle forms such as gatekeeping, controlling, or excluding.

Most champions did not share stories of horizontal violence. My experience was very different. Lots of peers bullied me over the years. It was usually subtle. Asking someone with lesser experience to deliver a workshop on a topic I was an expert in, not inviting me to lunches and morning teas, that general sense of exclusion you can identify much easier than you can articulate. Some have been more blatant. One peer made a formal complaint about me because I had expressed an opinion. It was public only because I replied to the same people in an email chain that she had and disagreed with her. It was a professional disagreement, an academic exchange, nothing personal. A couple of months later, I received a terse letter from my manager, a "please explain", advising me I may have breached the code of conduct. Seriously? For expressing an opinion. I was shocked. I believe that peer-to-peer bullying only occurs with the support of management. Even the university policy is clear that people with grievances should attempt to sort them out with the person concerned first. I'm positive had it been anyone else that process would have been followed. So basically, she handed them a knife to stick between my shoulder blades.

Peers bullied Alex from when she started her job. She believed they had it in for her. Even support from her manager did not stop their behaviours:

> Three women had an issue with me working there. When I started this job, one woman became extremely threatened by my presence. She was critical of everything about me, from what I ate and drank to my weight. She was critical of my intelligence and capability; she often insinuated that I was stupid. I did speak to her supervisor about it, and he tried to pull her in line and basically told her to pull her head in. She didn't, she just continued, and I tried to do the best I could. These women decided I was not wanted there and would do everything they could to leverage every bit of authority or power against me to oust me from that building at any cost.

Jordan described a particularly toxic individual who blatantly abused his position of power within the department to disrupt, harass, and intimidate peers he did not like:

> I worked with one of the biggest bullies I have ever seen. He would start with charm, and many people, including me, fell for that. When charm didn't work, the bully would emerge. He would raise his voice, and threaten with everything he could, even if it went beyond the bounds of his role. I remember when he took a dislike to a colleague. He started by patronising her, telling her she had to do better. She was running a very successful subject that boosted the numbers in the course he was coordinating. She was also a research student, and he was the coordinator of research degrees. He shouted in the corridor for others to hear that she better watch out because he would make sure she had a tough time. Outrageous. Sadly, this was not an isolated example. He did this all the time. Unfortunately, he got away with it.

3.5   Upward Bullying

She threatened to report me to the Vice Chancellor if I didn't retire (Jordan).

Jordan was the only champion who talked about upward bullying, bullying of managers by staff that report to them. I have experienced this too. Caroline came from an industrial background. She came across as very personable and very, very smart. Beneath it, she was one of the most conniving, manipulative people I had ever met. She was also very astute, reminding me of the scorpion in the story of the scorpion and the frog. She created this whole furore from what I believe was a minor incident. It certainly wasn't something that a mature conversation couldn't have resolved. Instead, she complained about me, and we were both called into a meeting with the head of school. I found myself facing accusations without warning. The Head of School barely allowed me the opportunity to respond and clearly showed her disgust when Caroline was giving her version of events. It was extremely badly handled. The head obviously heard one side of the story and took it as gospel. It was part of a culture that allowed that sort of thing to happen. Being dressed down by a staff member with my boss sitting there and providing implicit support was humiliating.

In Jordan's case, the bully was a student and casual health researcher. Jordan believed there were broader issues at play. However, the bullying was persistent and ultimately led to harassment and blackmail:

I was bullied by a PhD student who had also worked for me casually as a research assistant. She was experiencing stigma and discrimination more broadly. I did my best to be supportive and offered to go in to bat for her where it was appropriate. A pattern then emerged where I would somehow be placed in the role of the oppressor and put in the same category as the people who had discriminated against her or seen as responsible because I couldn't solve her issues. We would sort things out to a point and move on until the next time. It all erupted one night when I defended a person on a discussion list who had, in my opinion, been abused. I didn't even know him. The response from my student was, as I interpreted it, because of what had happened to her, I should just put up with this sort of thing. She dredged up everything she had previously complained about. I felt exhausted and let myself get caught up in a protracted email exchange. It went from there. She posted to the email group that I had refused to supervise her PhD. Although she didn't name me, it would have been obvious who she meant. It wasn't true, and I was disappointed she used a public forum to get back at me. She sent several offensive emails, the worst of which she copied to a long-term colleague. She threatened to report me to the Vice Chancellor if I didn't retire. Her last email was full of untruths. I replied and attached two emails that countered her version of events. Finally, I asked her formally and using very official language, with a hint of a legal tone, not to contact me again. I haven't heard from her since.

3.6   Mobbing

I was really mobbed. They thought they had permission to bully me … There would be no comeback. I was open game (Jesse).

Mobbing, the bullying of one or more individuals by a group, is sadly becoming much more common in health care and has profound implications for the target. Interestingly, this was one kind of bullying I didn't think I'd experienced. Reflecting a bit deeper, I was less sure. Understanding if mobbing has occurred again requires us to move beyond the common conception of bullying, often gained from our experiences of the schoolyard. Like all bullying, mobbing can include less obvious forms, such as stonewalling, excluding, and sabotaging reputations. I had been mobbed. I was heading a research centre. We shared our office space with another department. The arrangement was intended to be temporary, and it was made clear to me that I could organise the space to best suit the centre's needs. I wanted the research fellow to have his own office, away from the noisy open-plan area. I discussed room changes with my manager at least twice, and she agreed, but the people concerned didn't move. One woman was allocated an office in another building and told to move when she returned from leave. She came back and sat at "her" desk. She virtually had to be frog-marched out, and not before taking a computer monitor from right in front of a centre staff member, saying it belonged to her department, which was blatantly untrue. No point complaining. Nothing happened. When those staff finally left, they took everything that wasn't nailed down, including our fridge and microwave and most of the chairs. Despite being told nothing would be taken, I was admonished for complaining and told I should be grateful to have the space back.

Jesse, Alex, Taylor, Rory, and Terry all experienced mobbing. When Jesse became the target of her boss, her status was obvious to her co-workers, which gave them a *blessing to be mean*. Even colleagues she had enjoyed positive professional relationships with for several years became willing participants in her mobbing:

> I was really mobbed. They also thought they had permission to bully me, which is really off behaviour. There would be no comeback. I was open game. Someone else saw and said, what is happening? It was a very unpleasant scene.

What started as peer-to-peer bullying of Alex festered and grew to the point of mobbing. One co-worker had singled her out. When Alex began training as an Emergency Medical Dispatcher, her colleague had already spread her views about Alex to the educator and other trainees and influenced their opinion of her:

> I made a very bad assumption that once I was no longer working in that office, it would end, but it didn't. She had the educator there on her side, they're very close friends, and that's where it started becoming what I now know as mobbing. From the day we started, none of the other trainees seemed welcoming towards me.

While completing her training, Alex had to live on-site with her colleagues, who subjected her to bullying:

> It's a creepy building to be in at any time. I would come out to use the bathroom at night, and there would be nothing but black; there were laser images projected all over the walls and loud music playing. At times, some of them would come out and scare me as I went to the bathroom.

Alex found the strength to complete her training and looked forward to beginning her new career in a more positive environment, but unfortunately not to be:

> I was put on a roster with people that were very friendly and cosy with the boss, and it was an absolute nightmare. Every shift, these people tried to keep me from taking my breaks, even bathroom breaks. If I got up for an unexpected toilet break, I would have people follow me into the bathroom and question what I was doing. It's an experience that I still to this day reflect on, and I think how did I rationalise some of this for so long. But I did.

Taylor spoke up when she saw a nurse treating a patient disrespectfully. Defending patient rights was part of her role as an advocate, and it made her a target:

> It started with the first thing I saw that wasn't respectful towards one of the patients, and I raised it with that nurse, and that started it. You only have to get one nurse off-side and end up with all nurses off-side. There's one thing that nurses do pull together for, and that's when they're against someone.

Rory found herself unpopular with a consultant, an apparent personality issue. Unfortunately, the consultant had enough power and influence to set off a series of events and behaviours with other key staff in the organisation, which eventually led to Rory losing her job:

> I had a contract for a year but intended to stay longer if everything went well. Everything was going fine until a consultant came back from leave. I didn't understand that she was one of the Directors of Training, and she took an immediate dislike to me. Not in a way that I felt I needed to do anything about. We just didn't click. I don't need everyone to like me. When we started discussing rotations, I felt like my supervisor was saying one thing to me. This other person said: "How could you think you're getting that rotation?" and implied I was being really selfish. I felt very uncomfortable like I'd stepped on toes I didn't mean to. I moved rotations for a term and didn't love the culture in the new rotation. There were a group of consultants who didn't like or respect each other. I was put in many tricky situations, trying to manage their expectations and how I was meant to behave. There were a couple of little things that happened. I got more exhausted towards the end of the rotation. I got a bit snappier and more agitated at people being obstructive. My first assessment was fine, and the second one was less good, but none of them I thought were terribly bad, and the feedback was very vague. They just said I hadn't performed as well, and I said that I'd found this rotation particularly stressful. I was leaving. I didn't really want to go into it. Then, behind my back, they said all these nasty things about me to that consultant who didn't like me, and it just all snowballed from there. I had rotations removed, an upcoming contract shortened, and things taken away from me, and not told why. When I tried to ask for specifics and eventually made a complaint, it all got worse. Eventually, they didn't give me the contract at all. They offered me a job later in the year, so I temporarily moved away, but they retracted it as soon as I left. They told me it was due to funding. I called my previous mentor, and she told me that was a lie, and there were still positions available, but she had been told she wasn't allowed to speak to me. There were extraordinarily powerful people who no one wanted to cross. I had no ground to stand on because I was no longer an employee. And that's the problem with the whole medical model, that it's very easy to bully someone out by not giving them a further contract.

There was one specific incident when Rory was in the new rotation and trying to provide the best possible patient care. The incident was used as the catalyst to get rid of her:

> In one example that was used numerous times against me, I was referred a patient who was critically unwell and needed a dialysis catheter inserted. I just wanted the patient to get to the new unit so that I could do the catheter. In the end, I was like, okay, I'll go to emergency and do it there. One of the emergency department consultants walked in and said, "You can't do that here. You can do it in your unit". I turned around and said, really snappily: "I'm just trying to do the best thing for the patient". I picked up my stuff and left. I don't think a snappy comment where I'm just trying to do the best for the patient was enough to fire me. It was something that got used. I spoke to the director of my new rotation about it. He told me, "Don't worry about it, just leave it. You don't need to do anything". I was never spoken to about it until it was used against me. I think they were looking for reasons to justify something they wanted to do to me.

After experiencing bullying as a student and finding the culture in mental health services distasteful, Terry pursued an academic career. He thought the environment would allow for more freedom of expression. He could comment with authority on poor practices and be respected for voicing opinions and concerns. During his largely satisfying career, he started a new job, a joint position between a university and a health service. Unfortunately, the very structure and organisation of the role contributed to an environment where he felt mobbed by many of the staff he was expected to work collegially with:

> When I came here, I thought there would be resources. I thought there would be collaborative partners interested in going the extra mile in this project, and I found out that there's resistance built into the whole idea from the key people I would need to work with. The bullying started when other power struggles were taking place within the organisation. In particular, the consultants came under pressure to give up offices and wanted the funding for themselves. There were stories that started around me using hospital money and donations that could have gone to other parts of the service. I couldn't stop those narratives because I don't go to meetings in the same place as consultants. That's when life in the corridors became a nightmare.

It didn't end there. Terry's understanding of the research he would conduct before accepting the position differed from what the service wanted. He felt pressured to conduct research in areas where he didn't have the expertise or interest:

> The brief was to develop community-orientated models of service delivery, and what I'm asked to do is to help them reduce the levels of coercion inside the hospital. That's exactly the opposite. Had I been told I was expected to do a project on reducing coercion in the hospital, I would never have considered coming here.

His job soon became complicated to navigate without a consistent and clear vision for the role, differing expectations, and disappointment when Terry was not informed and therefore did not meet expectations.

It is very complex, and it took me years to figure it out because nobody told me what was going on. I've got a funder interested in doing good for the community. The clinicians will start asking for what they think would be good to have implemented, which will be different to what the funder envisions. Everybody will, at some point, start to speed up the process and ignore differences to get the whole thing up and running. And what I've come to realise now is that people were promised stuff that wasn't what I was asked to come here to do.

The outcome was that Terry felt bullied by many people within the organisation. He felt more like an intruder than a valued colleague:

I didn't want to meet people in the corridor because I knew people I said hello to would walk past me without a flinch and ignore me. My being, my physical being, can be ignored when I meet people in the corridors, so I am flat-out afraid of going there.

3.7   Beyond the Workplace

It's such a competitive, toxic environment, especially when you're not one of the gang (Jordan).

For some champions, bullying was also part of their professional work, including committees, professional organisations, volunteer work, and other activities related to their profession more broadly. In my experience, and it causes me great sadness to say this, professional organisations are full of competitiveness and self-interest, with so many big egos in one place. These organisations start with the very best intentions about strengthening the profession and bringing together like-minded people who want to make a difference. Unfortunately, it can quickly be a lot about people advancing their careers and increasing their profiles. Not all members behave this way. Unfortunately, many people who get actively involved in committees and take on roles like conference convener are in this boat. I have found horizontal violence to be extraordinary. Most of all, it wastes talent and energy that could be directed towards doing something constructive.

Jordan also described a highly competitive environment where personality issues prevailed over the organisation's best interests. She was not part of the clique and believed that certain people in power wanted her gone with bullying as their primary tool:

It's such a competitive, toxic environment, especially when you're not one of the gang. The professional organisation I'm a part of dealt me some of the worst bullying in my career. This is stuff people do in their spare time. It is bad enough being bullied at work. At least you get paid. The worst I've experienced was when a new chair came onto the organisation's Board. She and the director were very tight. There had been several issues with the director in previous years, and sadly they hadn't been handled well. The director was a bully. She was nice as pie when anything was going well, but when she felt her wings were clipped, she would become very oppositional and rude and worst of all, she would ignore the requests and directives of the Board. The new chair must've been like a dream come true to her. So many changes made were like a shopping list from the director. Unfortunately, I wasn't popular with either, and getting rid of me was one of their biggest priorities. One example - I had put a lot of work into a position paper that was approved by the previous Board. It was torn apart. I was more concerned about the other people on the subcommittee who had contributed to that work, only for it to be belittled and disregarded. It would have benefited the organisation. There may have been some issues that needed to be sorted, but to throw the whole thing out? It went from there. Anything I said or did was opposed.

Taylor had similar experiences. She left one committee because members did not consider her contributions, and she could no longer support and be seen to support the committee's business. Yet, she remained regretful and uncertain about whether she had done the right thing:

I stepped off a committee last year. It was important, important work. I stepped down because of the way the chair was treating me. They would not record minutes the way they should have. They were recording them in a way that made the committee look good, and they would not record my concerns, the things I asked for, or the things I wanted to be done. In the end, I left. It's the first time I've ever done that. I usually stay on and fight because I'm not fighting for me. I'm fighting for the human rights of people. I stay there, fight, or dance off these egos to try and get things done. But whatever I did, they were blocking. And I could not be seen as being a part of that. While I stayed there, they could tick the box that they had lived experience involvement. I'm so upset and now think I shouldn't have stepped down. Without my voice there, nothing will be achieved for people with mental health issues. I was really conflicted. If my suggestions and opinions had been respected, we, all of us, including people with mental health issues, families, carers, clinicians, and the community, would have benefited. But they would not listen; worse, they were prepared to falsely represent what I was saying.

Taylor was disappointed to have found herself caught up in self-interest and competition between peers in broader professional activities. She had been at the receiving end of some experiences that affected her career and the work she could potentially have done in a more collegial environment:

A couple of prominent advocates in the movement have caused me great pain over the years. But worse than this, they have not enabled the best outcomes we could have if we had worked closely together. If they had been gracious, had a generosity of spirit and were inclusive of me and other advocates I know have suffered, what could we have achieved? This lack of opportunity to do the best for our community hurts the most. A few people have stifled or even choked our good work over the years, and it's all about patch protection. At the behest of these people, I have been blocked from important conversations, left off important emails and invitations, and blocked from important positions on committees and councils that could lead to great improvements for our community. This led to blocking the advancement of my career at different stages. These people would say degrading things about me to people in influential positions. When I've been suggested as a Board member or something similar, these "advocates" already in the scene would say such things as "she is a show pony". That has completely derailed my career trajectory for a long time. I am so sad that we will never reach the full potential of what we could have offered our community if we had worked graciously together.

Jordan described the incestuous nature of professional organisations where it was more important to be liked than to be skilled or qualified for a particular role:

> It's like that saying, "It's not what you know; it's who you know". In this case, it doesn't matter whether you're an expert in a particular field. If they're looking for a keynote speaker or someone to join a committee, they are much more likely to go for someone who is one of them, a friend, a member of the gang or at least someone that doesn't threaten their egos. I've seen it happen time and time again. It's gone way too far when people cannot separate what is actually good for the organisation or the event from their own senses of who's in and who's out of the clique.

Shannon was bullied when working as a volunteer. She was seen to be "taking sides" by people witnessing her dealing with an incident, and some behaviours towards her changed:

> I volunteer for a church, and we make a homeless and disadvantaged lunch. There was an incident where a lady stabbed a man with a fork at a table. I just bounced into action. Mental health nurse, risk, let's clear the scene, let's make sure everyone's safe, everyone can move away, I've got you under control, frog march you out the door. And it was funny because I didn't realise the impact that had had on some of the other members at the lunch, and they saw me taking sides. After that event, I got a bit of bullying from some of the blokes, the big burly blokes. Just sexually inappropriate stuff that they'd never said before, and it was atrocious stuff. I had to get other staff around me to say they couldn't come back because they were so disgusting.

3.8   Recognising Bullying

> I just thought I was unlucky that I worked with a bunch of arseholes (Jordan).

Given it had taken me so long to recognise negative experiences as bullying, I wanted to know if this was similar for others. Like me, it took time for most champions to realise they had been bullied. Many incidents were seen as just the bad luck of working with unpleasant people, as Jordan and Sam talked about:

Jordan: Honestly, it took me the best part of 25 years to recognise it as bullying. I had this image of bullying as the stuff that happens at school. That wasn't my experience at work. It was much more subtle. When it happened, I just thought I was unlucky that I worked with a bunch of arseholes, people who felt threatened or were overly competitive, or whatever their reasons. I look back now and think, how could I have been so blind?

Sam: I didn't think of it as bullying for a long time. I thought it was just a person. And then, as various structures changed in the organisation, the bully became my senior nurse. That's when I was being told things in a corridor, I can't shortlist nurses for jobs anymore, or I can't do this anymore, or that is not my role, being left off lists. And despite my new boss speaking to the executive director, nothing changed. Two or two and a half years ago, I recognised it was bullying. Plus, it was pointed out by others that work for me they felt that I was denigrated or my position was denigrated.

Chris had worked in a particularly toxic organisation where the bully targeted several staff members. Although very unhappy about what was happening, there wasn't a clear understanding that they were bullied:

I didn't experience bullying myself. None of it was targeted at me. The person who did the bullying really valued me. People left because of this person's behaviour, and it took me a while to understand. If this person didn't like someone, if they had it in for them, then the person really made their life difficult and had the position to do that. The staff spoke about it a bit, but even then, none of us sat down and said, "This is bullying. This is what's going on".

Taylor believed many people did not see what was happening to them as bullying:

I don't think people do recognise what it is. They just see it as a problem. don't realise there are legal terms that it could and should be couched in. I didn't know about bullying or intimidation, or harassment. So, I never called it out in those terms.

Blatant and obvious forms of bullying were more likely to be recognised; subtle types often went unnoticed until they became an established habit. Shannon knew instantly she was bullied the first time. The more insidious behaviour in her recent experience had taken much longer to identify:

The first time, definitely, Instantly, once I got my head around it and realised who, what, and where, it was bullying. This time, it was more underhanded and hidden. It was very well manipulated, without us realising.

The misfortune of being bullied several times made it easier for Chris to recognise what was happening to her:

Over the years, I have gotten better at identifying what behaviour is what. When I had that first experience, I don't think I even really knew to formulate that this was workplace bullying. I just knew that she was horrible, and I didn't want to work with her. Looking back now, I can clearly articulate all the behaviours that constitute workplace bullying. I knew the behaviours weren't great. I knew that some people were treated differently. At the time, I didn't use the label of bullying. I never added it all up in my brain, until my experience, with that same person six years later. This person's behaviour changed towards me when I started to say, "This is not okay", when I pointed to inconsistencies in communication. I would try and have everything documented. Once this person realised that I was no longer an asset, the person embarked on a mission to get rid of me. And I'm like, "Oh, that's right, I remember this now; I've seen this before. I know what we're dealing with here. This is not good news". By that stage, I'd learnt much more about bullying. I'd done much more reading and was much more educated about it. So, I knew some of the behaviours were not okay.

Sam loved her work and wanted to make a difference; she wasn't interested in career progression. However, being so focused on the job at hand may have made it harder to recognise bullying until the senior nurse wouldn't allow her to manage staff recruitment:

I am not interested in ladder climbing. I wasn't really thinking about it other than it was hampering my ability to do my job. I suppose I was thinking, just send me the fricking email. If you send me the email, I can action it. Then putting together the whole hospital redesign, it became obvious to me because I was allowed to do the architecture, I was allowed to do the model of care, and all of those things. Then when it came to recruiting staff, I wasn't allowed to do that because I didn't have the qualifications. That's when it hit that this is not right.

Bully Tactics

4

The boss sent me to other centres … so I could learn to do my job properly, the job I'd already been doing for 20 years. I was horrified. I was absolutely humiliated (Andy).

In the previous chapter, the champions talked about how long it had taken to realise they had been bullied. A first step in addressing workplace bullying is to recognise it by understanding the different types of workplace bullies and their tactics, particularly the subtle ones. Gary and Ruth Namie, authors of "the bully at work", identified four main types of bully:

1. The screaming mimi
2. The constant critic
3. The two-headed snake
4. The gatekeeper

In my own journey to understand bullying, I found this helpful. Except for the screaming mimi, I could see many bullies in the other three. After the first two conversations with the champions and my first draft of this chapter, the constant critic didn't quite fit with these experiences. Criticisms of the champions were usually much more subtle than direct attacks on their credibility and reputation. Instead, I chose the term 'the saboteur' to describe this group of behaviours.

As we know, people don't fit into neat boxes, and bullies are no exception. All approaches to type or classify groups of people according to specific characteristics will be imperfect. Bullies may exhibit characteristics of more than one type and may alternate between them, sometime in a matter of seconds. Many people who bullied me could appear as a saboteur one day, a gatekeeper another, and quite possibly the two-headed snake most of the time. Tactics used against the champions related to all four bully types are the focus of this chapter, and there was no shortage of examples for each.

© The Author(s), under exclusive license to Springer Nature Switzerland AG 2024
B. Happell, *Sickness in Health: Bullying in Nursing and other Health Professions*, https://doi.org/10.1007/978-3-031-49336-2_4

4.1   The Screaming Mimi

> She starts pulling, tugging, violently shaking me. She is screaming uncontrollably at me ...
> I don't understand why this woman is attacking me (Alex).

When we think about bullying, the screaming mimi usually comes to mind. Screaming mimis are more like the bully we knew at school. They tend to be loud, aggressive, abusive, and potentially violent. They are obvious. Screaming mimis stamp their authority through overt and public criticism to make people scared of them. Scared people are easier to control. They scare the person they yell at and send a powerful message to others who witness it, "this could be you".

Alex was targeted by an educator at her workplace. She was abused, threatened, and physically attacked. The assault took her entirely by surprise and left her shaken, bewildered, and feeling unsupported:

> She got extremely agitated at my presence. We were on a break, and she grabbed me. She nearly knocked me over the railing. She starts pulling, tugging, violently shaking me. She is screaming uncontrollably at me, and I'm still trying to steady myself. I don't understand why this woman is attacking me. I don't understand why nobody's helping me. People are watching; nobody's doing anything. I kept saying, "Please stop. You're hurting me. Stop". She dragged me to another part of the campus, abusing me and screaming. I was cornered in a room with this woman attacking me, and there was nothing I could do but tell her I would speak to her at another time. That seemed to pacify her enough to let me out of the room. I reported the event, but it wasn't that day; I was shaken. I've never had anything like this happen, not even in my personal life.

Alex worked in a culture where screaming mimis were clearly tolerated, and she often found herself a target. She was ridiculed and humiliated by colleagues publicly, even when she engaged in her work:

> I had injured my wrist, and as I was coming into the room, she said, "Hey, have you been self-harming?" Everybody erupted in laughter. It was always at my expense. I was always the joke of that room, mimicking my accent and talking about my weight. It was relentless. The girl who emptied the trash one night – I will never forget as long as I live – I was on a call trying to help a patient in a horrible situation. She picked my trash can up, shook her head and said, "It amazes me the things people put in their mouth when they don't need to".

Taylor was bullied by screaming mimi colleagues frequently. She was verbally abused, had her property vandalised and received death threats:

> I would be yelled at and told I was useless. One doctor and some nurses would yell or say with clenched fists: "This is the mad leading the mad, and there's no place for you here". That I should be in a straitjacket instead of getting a pay packet. They also questioned the value of my work and my motive. That I'm only there for myself, for my own therapy. That I'm of no value. That my wage could be paying for another nurse's wage. My tyres were slashed. I'd get pieces of paper pushed under my office door with death threats. I got death threats on the phone. I got my nose tweaked several times by a doctor who had pinned me in a corner, yelling a tirade of abuse. He turned the entire staff against me and demanded that I be sacked.

Fortunately, most champions were not physically assaulted or threatened by screaming mimis. Instead, yelling and using abusive language tended to be their favoured tactics. Terry was verbally abused because the differing and unrealistic expectations in his job left him unable to conduct the research he was funded for:

> I couldn't get any traction to do the research I wanted to. I didn't have any places to implement the research, so I couldn't spend any money. The head of the funding department yelled at me. She really turned hostile towards me. I think it was out of frustration that I couldn't give her what she needed. I've tried to avoid her since because she was yelling at me and calling me a lot of really, really bad things. I ended up just getting up and saying "goodbye" and left, and I knew that I would never work with or trust her again. There is a complaint against her now. Finally, someone had the guts to say that she's abusive.

By their nature, screaming mimis make very clear their expectations that staff support them and their management style unconditionally. Questions and differing opinions are not tolerated. Lee often witnessed her boss publicly yelling at and intimidating staff and was often singled out herself:

> She screamed at the general manager in front of 20 of us in a meeting. She put up a PowerPoint depicting all the people who were happy about her changes as lovely people sitting around a table. Then there was a series of photographs of animals, a skunk, a sloth or a pig. All animals that people don't usually choose to be. "If you're not on board, if you're just about yourself, you're something else". One day, she called me into her office and said, "You're either with me or against me". I kept saying, "I'm talking about the issues. I'm not going to get into this". She screamed at me: "You're not with me, it's despicable, and I know about people conniving behind my back". I said to her, "You're losing it". She was red in the face, spitting, carrying on. "Let's end this here. You need to calm down. You need to not say the shit you're saying".

Chris was also yelled at and verbally abused. She described the bully as very clever, drawing short of making direct threats knowing too well what she could and couldn't get away with:

> There was never anything physical. There was yelling inappropriately at staff in front of people. But there were never any verbal threats. This person's not silly enough to do that sort of stuff. I remember having clinical supervision throughout all this and saying, "It just constantly feels like you're being drawn into a game of chess, where you know the person is already ten moves ahead of you".

Chris gave an example of the aggressive posturing and interactions used to intimidate her. Despite her shock, she was slightly amused that anyone in a leadership role would behave that way:

> One day I walked in the front door, and it almost looked like she was waiting for me. She said, "oh good; we've got tasks for you". It was almost like she was trying to stop me from interacting with others, and her physical posturing was puffed up chest, and that look on her face of, "Oh, don't mess with me. This is where your office is, so you get in there now and do those tasks we want you to do". And I had to stop myself from laughing because I almost couldn't believe someone could behave like that.

Sam was insulted and shouted at by the screaming mimi in a public place where other people could easily have overheard:

> I've done recruitment for all wards for 10 years. A year ago, she told me I was no longer capable of short-listing for positions and that she would do it. She screamed at me on the staircase.

4.2   Subtle Bullying

> It's what you can't see coming that will sideswipe you (Taylor).

No one will miss the screaming mimi, and whether the behaviour is recognised as bullying, it is obvious this person will be challenging to work with. It is not so easy for the other three types. The bullying is much more subtle. Taylor described subtle bullying as more dangerous and damaging because it was unexpected:

> You can see the obvious, prepare and take note of it, but it's what you can't see coming that will sideswipe you. That frightens me more.

Using subtle tactics was very powerful for bullies. They had an out, an option to dismiss behaviours as unintended, an oversight. This tactic worked well for Sam's senior nurse. When her boss attempted to confront the behaviours, the "sorry it was not intended" card was used:

> It is not her screaming at me in public and calling me a loser. It is insidious. Every time my boss has gone in there furious, saying we can no longer tolerate her behaviour, she will come up with an excuse, "Oh, I'm so sorry. I didn't realise that I had done that. It was not intentional".

4.3   The Gatekeeper

The gatekeeper uses bullying to control targets and influence their capacity to do their job effectively. These tactics include withholding information and resources, stonewalling, and exclusion. Gatekeepers create stressful environments that make it difficult, if not impossible, for targets to do their job at the standard they could without the obstacles. Most champions had an experience with gatekeepers, sometimes from one or a small number of people, other times from organisational units and teams. Some gatekeepers had recognised authority positions, while others were relatively junior.

Withholding Information

> I wouldn't find things out even when they were critical to patient care … I clearly wasn't important enough to know (Andy).

This is such a powerful weapon. It gives the bully so much control without saying a word, and it happened to me often. In one of many examples, I was misinformed and later left uninformed about recruitment processes. A staff member from my centre retired, and my boss told me there was someone at the hospital we could recruit immediately. My boss suggested I give her a three-month trial. I did. I wasn't happy with her and wanted to advertise the position externally. My boss was supportive and asked Frances, one of her staff to get the process in train. I heard nothing for a while, and I literally bumped into Frances in the tearoom and asked how it was going. I caught her off guard, "because you have someone in the position, you can't advertise for anyone else". I was horrified because this had never been explained to me, and she obviously had no intention of telling me. My boss initially said that was rubbish. I only needed to consider her for the position. She obviously found out otherwise down the track. I was told I would have to performance manage her for 3 or 4 months. I was shattered. My boss turned it around on me and said I should have known this, even though no one told me, and it was not the process I had been used to. Most of all, it was not what she had told me herself. It was a favourite tactic of hers to make it all my fault.

Shannon was the target of gatekeepers withholding information when she commenced a new job. She and her colleague were not adequately oriented to the role. Shannon saw this as a deliberate strategy to prevent them from becoming confident and competent in their roles and keep the bullies in power. One bully controlled the flow of information so successfully that she had become the central gatekeeper within the organisation, with staff, including those at senior levels going to her for information:

> These two young staff were training us. Both of us were mental health nurses with significant experience. They trained us with the bare minimum of information to be able to do our jobs to a basic standard. And it set up this amazing power play we didn't realise we were part of. We were constantly asking questions after seven months. Constantly not knowing stuff. We were part-time; they were full-time. So, things change on the day I'm not there, and no one tells me. I processed a referral, but, no, I can't send that referral to that organisation because they're full. No one told me. I'd constantly make mistakes, and they constantly went to the manager who said, "You've made another mistake". "I'm sorry. It's not a mistake. I wasn't aware of that". It's that knowledge is power thing. So, we did our work to the best of our ability, and then the other girls, in a senior meeting, just stripped us down, "This is crap. This is nothing like what we do. No wonder you guys make so many mistakes. You don't know what you're doing". There's a whole organisation above our heads, and every single person with a question goes to the head bully and asks her for everything. And she whinges, "Why does everyone come and see me?" "It's pretty easy, Diane. You really want to know?"

Timely communication has become an essential aspect of meeting work expectations effectively. Therefore, not responding to emails and messages becomes a powerful weapon for bullies to manipulate their targets. Many champions faced this regularly, making it difficult to successfully undertake their work roles. This was a persistent problem for Sam:

She doesn't answer my emails or texts unless I cc somebody in authority. I would email her, "Can you please put me on the agenda for the Nursing Managers' meeting so that I can talk about the new policy for 15 minutes?" No answer. Nothing. Then I would text and say, "I've sent you an email about such and such". No answer.

Lee accidentally discovered that information about conferences and other activities was not being circulated. Staff often missed hearing about conferences and events where they could present their research:

She would keep us out of the loop in terms of information and organise for herself to attend meetings. We were doing this clinical trial. In virtually every other place, the person in my role would attend these meetings. These trials were incredibly well-funded. There would be international trips in business class, and suddenly this woman would be going. She was getting the paperwork sent through her. It was only at local trial meetings, or we got something sent to everyone, or you get an email going, "Hope you're all recovering from Paris". I think Paris? "What's Paris?" And then you find out, oh, my God, for two months, she kept all the paperwork. You didn't know you weren't part of the system.

Andy found herself outside the communication loop. Even information affecting patient care wasn't conveyed to her, and she would often only find out about new procedures or processes when she came across them at work:

I wouldn't find things out even when they were critical to patient care. The information didn't trickle through. "Oh, you don't know that because you're only two days a week, we just didn't get to tell you". There's always an excuse, a cover-up, a reason. But you knew. You knew. Even the information that we were going to do this new procedure, I never knew anything about it. Suddenly, we are doing this procedure. You need to be specifically trained. The companies would fly people to Sydney, teach them about the procedures, and then supervise them. She could have asked me, "Do you want to work another day?" There wasn't even that conversation, let alone any conversation, about what was going on because I clearly wasn't important enough to know.

Withholding Resources

They never gave me control over my budget or expenses ... I couldn't buy a printer. I was completely disempowered (Terry).

Withholding resources effectively undermined the autonomy and authority of the champions' roles and became a significant barrier to work performance. Once again all too familiar to me. I was the head of a research centre, and suddenly when a new senior nurse started, I wasn't allowed a copy of the centre's budget because I wasn't officially an employee. I offered to sign a confidentiality agreement. No! I was told very firmly that it was policy that only employees could have these documents. Their compromise? I could look at the budget if I came to the pre-scheduled meeting with the senior nurse and the finance manager. Unfortunately, those meetings were held monthly, so I could be expected to wait for up to a month to see my budget.

Terry found himself in similar situations. He had accepted a senior-level academic appointment on the understanding that it would be an autonomous and well-supported role. Instead, he quickly found it quite the opposite, with no information or ability to access his budget.

> Everything around the hospital has been outside my control. They never gave me control over my budget or expenses. Never gave me insight into my accounts. I've been kept out of the loop completely. I've never been able to say I want to attend this conference because I've had no insight into what money is there. The only times I could spend money was if I said I needed this person to work with me two days a week, then I could have that person employed. I couldn't buy a printer, I was completely disempowered, so it's pretty outrageous.

Jordan ran a research centre with no administrative support after her assistant left. Her requests for help were denied, leaving her no option but to do the tasks herself:

> I was stunned by the total absence of support or assistance. It takes a lot for me to ask for help. I usually get on and do things. At one point, I needed help. I had no admin assistance and was organising a symposium on my own. I got nothing, absolutely nothing. I asked the senior nurse, who was saving salary if I could please have some assistance from her department. She said, "I'll do what I can, but I'm very reluctant to ask busy people to do more". Really? So, what are you doing now? Who else is going to do it? It was okay for me to do more, obviously. The research director at the university offered nothing. I asked him, "How would you manage without your assistant?" He went on about how wonderful she was and how he didn't even have to ask her to order tissues. They would automatically appear once they had run out. Thank you. That's brilliant. He never said, "Can I give you a couple of hours a week of her time? Anything would have made a world of difference to me. So, here's me, stuffing conference bags at home a couple of nights before the event, printing programs, and photocopying. I was doing everything somebody else could have done much more efficiently at half the cost.

Blocking

> One of my KPIs was to get 500 bums on seats at my webinar, but it was very hard to promote because she wouldn't sign off on stuff (Lee).

The champions were committed to their jobs, working hard, and achieving positive outcomes. Unfortunately, they were often blocked. For example, Sam's request to reclassify her position was blocked by the inaction of a bully. It had been for nine months at the time of our first conversation:

> We had a restructure, and my role changed. So, I've asked my senior nurse for a reclassification. I went through the process. My boss agreed that I met the criteria, so I submitted a reclassification form. This was last June. The procedure requires 14 days to respond. It's now March, and I am still waiting. When I send emails to my boss asking where we are up to, he sends them to my senior nurse. She either doesn't reply or with something like, "I'm reviewing her position". She's just ignoring my reclassification. It's bullying.

Part of Lee's performance evaluation was measured by people's attendance at webinars. The bully would often not provide approval for advertisement. Lee felt unable to take the matter further for fear of retribution:

> I ran a national series of webinars, and the bully was in charge of the communications department. They were terrified and wouldn't do anything without her. I wanted to advertise the program well ahead of time. "Oh, we have to have professional photos taken of people". I was organising that, and she wouldn't sign off on it. We couldn't advertise. One of my KPIs was to get 500 bums on seats at my webinar, but it was hard to promote because she wouldn't sign off on stuff. It wouldn't go into the newsletter. It wouldn't go on the website. She would say, "I'm pulling that because I don't like the language", but wouldn't say what she didn't like. If you didn't have any disturbances with her, this wouldn't happen. A couple of our webinars went out with literally no advertising. On the day, only 50 people subscribed. Some staff were livid because even though there were many explanations, no manager wanted to hear the minutiae of that: "Well, how come only 50 people came to this webinar?" "You were getting 400 or 600 signing up, or even 800. What about this?" I had grounds I could complain, but if she knew she was questioned, there would be other ways of cutting off your head and making life very difficult.

Micromanagement

> The manager sat me at a desk right outside her office, and it started ... In the first week, I got over 60 emails about what I was doing that she didn't like (Pat).

Micromanagement, as the name suggests, describes the bully closely monitoring the target's work to the point that innovation and productivity are stifled. Shannon and Jordan talked about their experiences of micromanagement:

Shannon: Those two junior staff oversee our work. They go back through our completed referrals and check them to make sure that they're up to standard.

Jordan: The senior nurse was on leave, and I was planning a trip interstate. I sent an email to the person acting. I provided details. I will attend meetings, supervise students etc. I gave an estimate of costs and said it would come from my consultancy account. This had always been a straightforward process. Her answer: "Happy to consider this further. Can you provide a little more background about how this is related to ongoing work you are involved in currently?" Holy crap, what difference would that make? Was there some decision I couldn't do anything new I hadn't been told about? No point arguing, so I provided a tedious amount of information. I reminded her the funds were coming from my own account. I must have jumped the necessary hoops, and the travel was approved. So, was she just particularly pedantic or being over-cautious? From my past dealings with her, I doubt it. I'm sure she was following instructions from the boss. Micromanagement became the order of the day from around that time. I suspect it was punishment for raising concerns about my relationship with the senior nurse. It was intended to be confidential, but clearly not.

Pat returned to work after an extended period of sick leave. She had previously enjoyed a collegial and autonomous role. In sharp contrast, the new manager closely monitored and criticised her:

> The manager sat me at a desk right outside her office, and it started. If I came into work of a morning and had my personal mobile phone, and I was turning that off, it was, "You're using your personal mobile too much". I said, "I'm actually not using it. I was turning it off and putting it into my bag". "Oh, well, you can't". So, I was emailed a copy of the policy for using personal mobile phones at work. In the first week, I got over 60 emails about what I was doing that she didn't like, and I thought, oh, this is not good.

Micromanagement is a sign of poor leadership. Lee and Jordan were used to autonomous positions, so the sudden hyper-vigilance and close monitoring of their movements left them feeling they were not trusted. It was like there was an underlying sense of a more significant issue that was playing out through indirect and passive-aggressive tones rather than being dealt with directly:

Lee: It's fascinating to go from a really open workplace where they just trusted you. If I said, "I've got a window guy coming, I'm working from home today", no one gave a shit, and I got all the work done, but suddenly, you're in this environment where they're like, "Well, what time will you be in? What time is the window man coming?" I'm going, "Have you ever dealt with a tradie? I don't fucking know" You felt you had to prove yourself. So, I would start doing stuff at 7.30 or 8 o'clock in the morning that I would email, so they knew that I was active because there was this complete lack of trust.

Jordan: I travelled a lot for work. That had never been a problem. Then, suddenly, the tide changed. No words were spoken, no concerns raised, just these passive-aggressive messages from the senior nurse: "Are you not at work this week? Your out-of-office says you won't be back till Monday". Clearly, she answered her own question. She had the nerve to ask if I was on annual leave or was there another purpose for my travel? Had she bothered to look, she'd have found that the acting senior nurse had approved the leave, and her PA had organised the trip. That passive-aggressive crap, as much as to say, "I'm on to you, I know you're lying to me". If that's what you think, why don't we have a conversation? Are we bloody adults, for fucks sake? You're the one with all the power. If you have a problem with me, have the decency and the professionalism to raise it with me. Some chance.

Exclusion

> One of the girls who seemed the most aggressive of the group, if I would raise my hand to ask a question, would actually tell me to be quiet (Alex).

One potent bully tactic I experienced on many occasions was exclusion. I was communicating with the research office as I was about to submit a large grant application and received the message that no staff would be available on a particular day. They were attending the strategic research day. I was a very senior researcher, one of only two professors at that level, and I was not invited. What possible explanation could there be other than not being liked and clearly not part of the plans for the future? I know my counterpart was there. I rang his office and was told he was unavailable, "at the strategic research day?" I asked. "Yes".

I was not alone. Exclusion from both work-related and broader social activities was a strategy champions frequently experienced when they were out of favour with a bully:

Sam: It's insidious. I'm excluded. There are nursing meetings I'm not invited to. I'm not included in emails, email lists, or professional nursing information. It's forwarded to me by the nurses I'm professionally responsible for. They will say, "Do you know about this?" Or they'd tell me they'd received an email saying I would no longer be doing their performance appraisal; it would be done by her.

Taylor: Not being asked to meetings where my voice was really important. Not getting notices, not getting minutes, not being invited to parties, discussions stopping when you step into a room and when you walk out of the room, laughter and conversations starting again. All the time.

Lee: The team wanted to put in a submission. Early on I'd had some things to say about it. After that, I wasn't invited to any meetings.

Terry was asked to be part of a funding application. He was actively involved in its development with an understanding that he would have a key role in the research. Instead, he received no resources and his input into the application was completely ignored. Despite his anger, he felt trapped and unable to make a complaint:

> I was tricked into being part of a grant application because they needed a token nurse. It was successful, and the other investigators took all the money, and I heard nothing. I don't know what to do because I'm really pissed off, and I should say go F yourself, but at the same time, the university system will punish me if I'm not an investigator on successful grants. My CV looks like I'm part of something, so I need to comply with a corrupt system. My contributions to the protocol have been ignored, and I'm completely ignored. I have nightmares about it. I'm not linked to any of the communication between anyone. Honestly, I was set up. He needed a nurse to indicate this was interdisciplinary. I had no idea that meant I had no influence on what would happen.

While often insidious, exclusion could also be blatant, as Alex experienced:

> One of the girls who seemed the most aggressive of the group, if I would raise my hand to ask a question, would actually tell me to be quiet (Alex).

Lee and Jordan often found themselves left out of social events other staff organised and attended:

Lee: I'd walk into the kitchen at lunchtime, and everyone else is eating
          Vietnamese. They've obviously gone out and got it or had an Uber Eats
          brought in, and, "You haven't invited me".

Jordan: The other staff would go out to lunch together; it seemed about every
          second day. If I were in my office with the door open, they'd walk right
          past. If I met them in the hallway, they would ask, "Are you coming for
          lunch?". "I'm too busy", I'd reply. Off they'd go, and not once did any of
          them ask if there was anything they could do to help.

4.4 Two-Headed Snake

Two-headed snakes are often tricky to identify because they appear supportive and collegial. The target usually becomes aware of the deception when the damage has been done. These bullies seek to control and even destroy their target's reputation under cover of collegiality or even friendship. Their behaviours include backstabbing, taking credit for the target's work, and playing favourites. Discovering bullying can be particularly distressing because a fundamental trust has been broken. I have often experienced this from peers in the workplace and my broader professional community. I've known colleagues who, behind a veneer of collegiality and mutual commitment to the broader profession, would destroy my reputation without hesitation. Fewer examples of two-headed snakes were described by the champions. However, I suspect many of the gatekeepers and saboteurs share these characteristics.

Backstabbers

> They know how to play the game … and look like they're saying and doing all the right things in front of other people. They have turned other people against me (Taylor).

At one place I worked. I was surrounded by backstabbers. Like many others with similar experiences, I didn't realise the extent of it until the damage was done. I ran a research centre which was funded or supported by a large group of stakeholders.. I copped it from all of them. Many key people were all smiles and encouragement. One in particular I had known professionally for a long time. She portrayed herself as direct and transparent. We met regularly and discussed plans and activities together. I thought we had an excellent professional relationship. But, boy, was I wrong? She and her boss totally shafted me and used the power of the funding to "move me on". There were many other willing participants, including my own boss. It came completely out of the blue, leaving me shattered. I had given my all to that job, achieved outcomes, and built a great team. All my performance appraisals had been outstanding, and then, wham.

Jordan discovered her boss was a two-headed snake at her performance appraisal. It became apparent that her view about their working relationship was not shared by her boss:

> I thought wc had a pretty good working relationship. We had our moments and felt we usually resolved them. She called a spade a spade, and I respected that in her. I had no reason to believe she wasn't happy with my work. I still have an email I received when I sent her our annual report. "It looks fantastic. Well done to you and the team but particularly to you. This reflects the work and the reputation the centre is developing under your leadership". Four months later, in my performance review, she absolutely shredded me. "Yeah, yeah, fine, you've done this, and you've done that, and you're good at this, and you're good at that, but you haven't done this, that and the other thing". And I was like, wow, where did this come from? She was totally hostile. Even how she sat, right at the back of the room, almost pushing her Chair against the wall, not around the table like she always had. Her arms were folded, and there was only fleeting eye contact. It was like a completely different person. I was blindsided. And after saying a few things in my defence that she abruptly dismissed, I didn't bother. I just sat there and listened. I was shattered when I left that room.

Terry believed he had a very supportive and open relationship with a colleague. He later discovered she had been presenting a very different picture to others and creating even more barriers to his job performance:

> She works at the hospital where I work, where she's been talking behind my back. Whenever I met her, she would say, "This is good. Let's try this. Let's do that". I heard through the back channels that she was talking badly about me, slowly making it impossible for me to penetrate the medical dominance in the hospital.

Two-headed snakes were particularly challenging when they held positions of respect and influence. Taylor described the actions of a colleague, a leader in the broader professional community and highly influential to others:

> Because they are so respected, I can't speak out about it. It just looks like I have sour grapes. They know how to play the game. They are the master of subtle destruction and know how to look like they're saying and doing all the right things in front of other people. They have turned other people against me and caused me immense grief.

Taking Credit

> It's not that you don't get your piece of cake. You don't even get the crumbs off the table. It's all about her, and it's just who she is (Jesse).

The two-headed snake Jesse worked with blatantly took credit for and reaped the rewards of work she had little to do with. Jesse's role was not acknowledged. She went along with this, believing she would ultimately be rewarded. Unfortunately, this was not the case:

> There were two of us in the program, but it was just her who got all the kudos. That didn't bother me so much, except after working for her for 10 years, she said, "I'm not going to

worry about making sure you have a job for next year. You're going to have to worry about that". So, I had no job. It's not that you don't get your piece of cake. You don't even get the crumbs off the table. It's all about her, and it's just who she is.

Favouritism

She would make it difficult if you opposed her for anything. You would be left out (Lee).

Two-headed snakes invariably have their favourites, often friends or sycophants, who help them feel secure in their role. Favourites get an easier ride and more praise. I've seen this a lot. In one job, it was blatant. The head of school took every opportunity to congratulate the deputy, who also happened to be her friend. Every paper she published was sent to the school with statements like "What a productive writer she is!" It would have been fine if the same practice had been applied to everyone, but it wasn't. Far more productive staff received far less attention. We had a colleague who was incredibly innovative with her approach to teaching. The media did a full-page story about her work in the local newspaper. I sent it to the head so she had no excuse to pretend she hadn't seen it. She sent it to the school and said, "Please find attached a newspaper snippet about Sonia". Snippet? I couldn't believe it. Her deputy would've got bigger coverage if she won a chook raffle. That's just one example: People from the inner circle got lighter workloads, less popular staff, and anyone who wasn't a friend worked much harder. It was so blatant. It showed what she thought about the rest of us. We'd have to be stupid not to see that.

Lee talked about the stark contrast between how the targets were treated and those the bully liked. Favourites received additional resources and promotions, while she and other targets didn't:

There were some people she liked who got credit, new titles, pay bumps, and anyone she thought was against her, she didn't do a thing for, or she belittled and ran down or bullied. They used to have an admin person two days a week. She was on board with the boss. She expanded her role to full-time. When we counted the emails that came in, this woman has had 30 emails this month, one a day, but 15 were just Zoom invites to a meeting. So, every second day, she has an email to deal with, and they've made her full-time. I could sit at my desk and see 15 come in within an hour, plus the phone's ringing and everything else.

It was clear to Lee that playing favourites was also an effective way of keeping the targets in check by punishing staff who didn't behave as expected. When challenged, the bully came up with excuses:

She would make it difficult if you opposed her for anything. You would be left out. Everyone else would be going to conference X or getting support for it. She would say to me: "Oh, well, everyone who is going to the conference has to have a presentation. You can't just go because you're interested". I'd say, "I put three papers in. I've got two accepted. I've got four posters". "Oh, well, somebody has to stay and do the trial".

In another workplace, Lee clearly saw the impact favouritism had on morale. Staff who did not align themselves with the bully suffered consequences. She talked about one experience where the entire team could not do their job effectively because of bullying. Being unable to work to her own standards, Lee ultimately decided to leave:

> If you didn't fall in line with her, there would be meetings you didn't get to go to, withholding information and being really difficult about basic things. It was just so difficult for me to do my work because there was mobbing and bullying, and there was just this difference in the way people were treated. Staff would be so upset and distressed that they'd be on sick leave, stress leave, or they would be there, but they'd be unable to focus on work. It just becomes exhausting in the end. That contributed a lot to my leaving. Life's too short to be getting people to check an email before you send it.

Jesse was also blatantly singled out for unfair treatment:

> I was at a status where everybody else had their own personal admin assistant. I got to share one with the pool. Everybody else at my level got new furniture in their rooms, but I didn't. He tried to stop me having a research career. He didn't give me enough time to do research and stopped me from doing projects. He restricted students that I could have, all these quite unfair restrictions that others didn't have.

4.5 The Saboteur

Most bullying the champions experienced was at the hands of the saboteur. The saboteur's end game is to destroy their targets' credibility and reputation. They achieve this by humiliating, undermining, attacking reputation, imposing unreasonable work demands, changing the goalposts and exploiting vulnerability. They strike the person's confidence and, ultimately, their perceived capabilities for their job.

Humiliation

> They call us out in front of everyone for stuff that we do wrong, but, in fact, it's not that we're doing it wrong. It's just that we've never been shown how to do it correctly (Shannon).

Nothing shatters a person's sense of confidence and self-worth more than humiliation. I remember feeling totally embarrassed by the actions of my boss. I was part of an international research consortium, and we were meeting face to face in Europe. I submitted the necessary paperwork and approval from the senior nurse to the acting dean. I advised that the meeting was required for all project team members and was funded through the project. Surprise, surprise, that wasn't enough. He actually asked me to provide evidence that I was required to attend. Really? I am in a senior position at the university and the hospital. I am involved in this project because of my international reputation as a leader in this field. I have to prove that I must be there! I had to ask the project lead to send me an email confirming that the meeting was a requirement. I know he was shocked. It was humiliating. I can't see any other reason for it than to belittle me. I suspect he would have said no if it wasn't a requirement. Imagine, "Oh, sorry, team I can't come to this meeting. I'm not allowed". One thing to belittle people privately, quite another when others bear witness.

Andy had been working at her current job for years when her boss told her to go to other similar centres to learn her job properly. She was expected to learn from peers holding the same level position. Andy was embarrassed and humiliated to be put in this position:

> The boss sent me to other centres to watch what other assistant managers do so I could learn to do my job properly, the job I'd already been doing for 20 years. I was horrified. I was absolutely humiliated. It was just the worst experience of my life. I told the other managers that my new manager had asked me to come along and see what processes you have in place to do the things that we do, to see if there is anything different. They knew.

Lee was humiliated when she was directed to lie to people who wanted to attend an event at the organisation for no reason other than the bully's desire to block people she didn't like:

> We were having a stakeholder event, and she made me ring up people who wanted to come and say, "Oh, we're full, but we'll put you on the waitlist". We weren't full. We didn't have enough people to come, but they were people she called troublemakers who had dissenting opinions from her; she didn't want to come.

Sam was accused by the bully of making a wrong decision in a meeting. However, it was clear the bully did not understand the circumstances and didn't bother asking or trying to grasp the reasons behind the decision:

> I went to this meeting, and she was saying we were wrong, "This girl should have been referred to the eating disorders ward. I'm not sure why you didn't do that". It was denigrating. I said that maybe we could have considered that. Because I didn't want to denigrate her publicly. My patient was 14 years old. The service she is talking about will not take anybody under 18.

Sam found it difficult to deal with public intimidation because she did not want to be seen to be retaliating or drawing others in. She found herself having to defend the bully to colleagues:

> She's publicly denigrated me on a couple of occasions, and that's been really difficult. Staff came to me and said, "Oh, my God, what have you done to her?" And I said, "I'm sure you misunderstood what was going on", because I acted professionally.

For Jesse, the humiliation was blatant and deeply personal:

> It got so bad that I was in a meeting, and I was asked a question. I responded, and I stutter a little, sometimes, and he actually laughed at me stuttering.

Shannon was already embarrassed when she was summoned to HR. She was devastated to discover the bully had told other staff she was "in trouble".

They were aware of what was happening to me. Because my manager brought it up in the team meeting that something had happened. I was heading off to HR, and that perhaps I might not return.

Chris was mortified by the organisation's response after submitting her resignation. She felt humiliated by their complete disregard for her and lack of consideration for the best interests of her clients:

When I handed in my notice, they said, "Thanks. You can finish today". I had no idea they would think about doing that to someone in a clinical role. I was devastated because, oh my God, I couldn't even say goodbye to my clients. Some I'd worked with for 2 to 3 years, and I don't know what they were told. I didn't get to handover to anyone. I couldn't even get my head around that they wanted me gone that badly. The impact on patient care, it was unbelievable. The day I went to hand in my work phone, I wasn't even allowed into the building. What has the bully said to make them feel that I'm not safe to walk in the building? I'd never been treated like that in my life and certainly hadn't done anything to warrant it.

Working at home during the COVID-19 pandemic did not protect Shannon from humiliation in front of others. She was angry that these toxic behaviours were now intruding into her home:

It's in a group, our video chats. They call us out in front of everyone for stuff that we do wrong, but, in fact, it's not that we're doing it wrong. It's just that we've never been shown how to do it correctly. I can't believe it can be so toxic, even in my home. And I'm really annoyed at that. Like, it's in my own home, get out of my home!

Undermining

They have undermined me … with my peers and my community. I still grieve what that relationship could have been … People say you can't lose what you never had. I actually think you can (Taylor).

When bullies undermine, they weaken the target's authority or position. When a new boss started, the little autonomy and respect for my role in the organisation quickly disappeared. A new clinical researcher was appointed. She came from overseas, and it took about 14 months from recruitment until she arrived. No office was organised. The research centre I was supposedly in charge of had three offices and six hot desks. The three full-time staff members occupied the offices, so I offered her a hot desk. I went to a meeting with her and the senior nurse. The senior nurse told me the researcher needed an office, and my assistant would have to move to a hot desk. I tried to discuss it, but it soon became evident that the decision had been made. The researcher clearly thought she was entitled to an office to suit her station, although she was half-time and supposedly spent most of her time in the clinical areas. My valued staff member was just an assistant who could sit anywhere. I don't think that way, so it stung. My assistant's office was directly opposite the front door, so she was accessible. She could see if people were trying to gain access to the locked area. She was moved around the corner. It is bad enough that it should happen at all and unforgivable that the senior nurse should do that to me in front of the researcher. That said everything about who was valued and who wasn't.

Sam found herself constantly having her authority challenged by her senior nurse in the presence or knowledge of others:

> People from the [health] department wanted to come and visit the ward and talk about the work that we do. So, I sent my senior nurse an email saying, "People from the department are coming out on this date. Please let me know if you would like to join us". She wrote back. "I will organise this. This is a job for my office". I said, "Okay. Please let me know what you'd like me to do?" She said, "I'll let you know what time you can come". But then, she had to include me because she knew nothing about the service.

Jordan felt totally intimidated when her boss "pulled rank" on her by making a decision without discussing it and framing it as being in her best interests:

> I was totally undermined by the dean. I had a casual research assistant working for me. She hadn't been meeting her goals. She sent her final pay sheet. I asked her to send the work she'd claimed to have done, and I would approve it. She accused me of bullying her, forcing her to undertake unnecessary flights on a business trip when she had chosen those flights and many other false accusations. So, my boss went in over my head and approved the claim. I was livid, and I told him so. He told me he was protecting me. From what? I haven't done anything wrong. I told him I could prove that what she was saying was untrue. He didn't care less. He wanted the problem solved, and making life difficult for me was a bonus.

Andy's boss tried many ways to intimidate her, often insinuating she was in trouble. On one occasion, she suggested Andy had taken too much leave, and it had been noted by HR:

> She said I had been red-flagged by HR for the amount of leave I took. So, I said, "Excuse me". She was trying to intimidate me, and I don't know what her end game was, but probably to make me leave.

Intimidation as a bullying tactic was not confined to the workplace. Taylor and Jordan experienced bullying from colleagues from their broader professional networks:

Taylor: This person and I have been colleagues, and I acquiesced to them a great deal of the time out of respect and fear. Out of respect because they have done the hard yards. The number of times they have undermined me in conversations with my peers and my community. I still grieve what that relationship could have been, should have been. People say you can't lose what you never had. I actually think you can.

Jordan: This Board I was a part of, the Chair always tried to intimidate me by positioning me as ignorant and her as all-knowing. We had an issue. A couple of emails went back and forth about who could and couldn't chair a working party, and I thought I'd ring her. It was a genuine desire to sort it out as adults. She made statements like "You must understand good governance". So, I said, "Okay, where is this written in any of our guidelines or our constitution?" I just got the same old "You must understand good governance". "And what's good governance? What you say it is?" If you're not prepared to support your statement with evidence, you're intimidating someone with your position. That's not how professionals should work, let alone health professionals.

Attacking Reputation

The educator had talked with the other new trainees about me. She was already poisoning the well with them (Alex).

Bullies sought to discredit champions' integrity and credibility to control how their colleagues saw them. They attacked the reputation of targets either directly or indirectly. For example, Lee was set up by her boss for apparently refusing to approve a leave request, resulting in an unhappy and disgruntled staff member:

One staff member was told I didn't want her to take leave, unbelievably untrue. I had approved someone's Easter leave in November before. The boss tried to cancel it and say that I didn't want them to have it and this person was shitty to me. I never knew why and then somebody said, "Oh, I think she's still shitty that you wouldn't let her have leave at Easter". I was, like, "The fuck?" So, we went through my files and forwarded her the email, and I said, "I supported it. I never said you couldn't".

Chris was unwittingly embroiled in a plan to set her up as a bully. Other staff were questioned about Chris and whether she had bullied them in what seemed an attempt to collect damning evidence:

I feel like they were trying to set me up for being a bully. One of my colleagues said, "I've just had a horrible experience". She felt that the bully was prying, fishing, and planting seeds saying, "Have you ever felt bullied by Chris?" She told the person categorically, "No. We have an excellent working relationship". She got on the phone to me because "I'm worried that they're going to try and accuse you of being a bully".

When Alex started her training, she discovered the educator had already tarnished her reputation and turned other trainees against her:

One of the gentlemen in my class told me that the educator had talked with the other new trainees about me. She was already poisoning the well with them.

Unreasonable Work Expectations

It's very subtle stuff. One piece at a time is nothing, but all adds up to a huge weight on your shoulder (Andy).

The champions and I could fill the book on this topic alone. One particularly annoying example was when my boss felt entitled to intrude on my annual leave time. She sent an email requesting information she needed to provide a report with a short turnaround. She said she realised I was on leave and hoped I was checking emails. Really? Shouldn't a decent boss be hoping I wasn't? That I was actually taking the break I deserved? I did what she asked promptly and sent it back. Things were bad enough between us without risking the fallout of ignoring her email. Back from her? Nothing, no thanks, no acknowledgement.

Lee found herself with a much heavier workload than many of her colleagues, which she believed was a deliberate attempt to bully her:

> I'm trying to do 100 hours of work in the 30 hours that I'm paid for. She increased other people's fractions. We have one program where the staff were very close to the bully. The woman managing the program, of about 200 instructors, I look after 2,200, had worked two or three days a week, and she was made full-time. They had a full-time person and a full-time admin person. So, a program of 200 people, 3 EFT, helping and supporting. I've been employed 4 days a week and manage all the other programs.

Lee was angry and knew she'd have been totally justified in refusing to take on all that work. But, at the same time, she felt obliged to get the job done for the sake of the organisation even though she would never expect the same from others:

> I was sent stuff on my day off. We had no staff. So, I did 500 hours of overtime because the whole ship would have fallen over if a couple of us didn't step up. I think maybe I shouldn't have. I should have just let them fucking fall apart. I come from a very stoic background, taught not to complain and to get on with it, and it's not about you. In some ways, that's great, but it also does us a great disservice. Managing someone else myself, I would have said, "You can't do it". "It's not reasonable", "Tell them no", and yet I've never done that myself.

When Jesse sought refuge from her boss by requesting a secondment to the university, he agreed, provided she completed an impossible workload beforehand. Jesse was very proud she completed the work and overcame his attempts to block her:

> I told him, "I'm going to take this 10-month secondment". He said, "Yeah, of course, you can, but you've got to finish this, this, this and this first". So, he gave me, in a two-week period, about three months of work to do before I could go. You should've seen his face when I did it. He didn't actually think that anyone could do it, and I did. When I left, they replaced me with three people.

Unreasonable demands were sometimes so subtle they were difficult to prove. Andy faced this. She had no doubt it was happening. It was often little things, not much on their own, but they added up to a lot more:

> If you looked from the outside, you couldn't probably see it. It's that kind of bullying when you go, "Oh, but I've been doing all the work". "Well, that's what you're here for". "Yeah, but not everyone else is doing all the work the same as me. Not everyone else is not getting the opportunity to be a clinical nurse consultant". Even when she was on holidays, she would have staff make sure that I was not rostered to have any time out of the lab. It's very subtle stuff. One piece at a time is nothing, but all adds up to a huge weight on your shoul-

der. We all got new led aprons to wear in radiation. Every single person got their name embroidered on them except for me. "Oh, it must have been an oversight". But there are constant examples. Nothing huge by itself, but every little thing. We have a trolley bay area and reception where the patients come pre-procedure and go back afterwards. I was the only person that worked 10-hour days. So, I would regularly work in the trolley bay because 10 hours is a lot in lead. That stopped, and I was never allowed to be in the trolley bay again. "Because you only work part-time, you can be in radiation all the time". Whatever lab was the busiest, that's where I went.

Unreasonable work demands weren't only dished out in the workplace. Champions working from home or otherwise out of the office were not immune from this form of bullying:

Lee: I'd wake up at 7 in the morning, and there'd be a message saying, "I want this, and I want it done now". We used to have a policy saying we would not contact each other outside 8 till 6, but she would scream at you from first thing in the morning.

Jordan: I had flown interstate for an evening meeting and a morning one the following day. I received an email at 6.30 pm with something like: "I understand you're interstate for a meeting, but your input is needed by tonight". The centre's research manager had been asked earlier that day to provide information about our research activities. He turned that around in just over 3 h to meet the university's deadline. The email comes from someone at the hospital, and let's not forget, I'm not an employee of the hospital. I sent her what was done. She sends an email to the research manager, who works for me and is also not employed by the hospital, at 7.00 pm asking for the information to be presented differently and in more detail by the following morning. I advised her that he would likely not access email until the next morning. We didn't do it within her ridiculous time frame. That was probably another nail in the coffin. Still, I wasn't prepared to be bullied into cancelling meetings and fulfilling unreasonable deadlines for an organisation that tells me I don't work for them as soon as look. I definitely won't let people who work for me be bullied.

Shannon and her colleague, both mothers of young children, faced unreasonable working conditions and a lack of consideration for their family circumstances while working from home during the COVID-19 pandemic:

We are the only people in the team that have children. We're the only people that are home-schooling. We were presented with a roster of our lunch breaks, with no discussion and a new roster, because one of them wanted to finish at 3.30 on a Friday. She wanted to work half an hour extra here and there, and I would have to work an hour later on a Friday afternoon. I wasn't asked. My lunch break was 1 o' clock, and I said, "Sorry, I can't do that. My children have a lunch break at 12.30". "That won't work with everybody else". I said, "Why? What are your commitments for your lunch?" The response was, "Don't make it too difficult". That's more than a reasonable request when you've got two of us with children and two without.

Changing the Goalposts

> The bully would do anything to get rid of me ... She knew what things were important to
> me, and she systematically took all those things away (Chris).

The champions frequently worked with bullies who constantly "changed the goalposts" with commitments, work roles, and expectations. For example, Rory's supervisor agreed to her having a rotation in a specialist area that was important for her career plans. That agreement was later withdrawn, and her supervisor denied everything:

> I had a supervisor that didn't respond to emails. So, everything was verbal. And then he
> denied it, even though we mapped it out on a piece of paper, and he showed me the roster
> on the computer. I wasn't manipulating things. I'm an honest person. If he had said it was a
> maybe, I would have known it was a maybe, but it wasn't.

Andy and Chris also talked about how the bully would tell them what they had to do and often later change their version of events:

Andy: She would say, "Do X, do Y, do Z". And I would do X, do Y and then she'd say, "No, I never said that. I asked you to do A, B and C, and now you've done everything wrong". For example, she asked me to see how we could work together and do a test to see what sort of personality you are. So, I found something and booked it, and she said, "I didn't ask you to do that. You're not allowed to do that. How dare you?"

Chris: Meetings being shifted, and things being agreed to, then reneged on. And then you'd go back and say, "This is what you said", "Oh, no, I never said that". So, then you look like an idiot in front of everybody else.

Chris was ultimately informed by HR that if she continued to do specific work, she would be in breach of her contract. Even though she had her boss's approval, her version of events was not believed:

> There were basically lies. I would meet with her one-on-one and say, "Can I have some
> clarity? Now that you're changing my role, am I able to do X, Y and Z?" She would say,
> "Yes, great". So off I'd go and start doing whatever, and then I'd get a letter from HR say-
> ing, if you continue to do this, you will be in breach of your contract. And I'm like, "I was
> just told by my manager two weeks ago that I could do that". "Oh, I'm sure your manager
> didn't say that". So, I was made out to be the liar, making things up and stirring trouble.

Changing the goalposts created considerable uncertainty and anxiety for Andy. She had no idea what might change next and knew there was a good chance she would be blamed for the outcomes:

> We had set up a clinic at our centre where patients came into us because we had such an
> experienced wound care nurse. We had a launch and Members of Parliament, GPs, every-
> thing. Our head office was all over it, loved it. She told me to stop giving referrals to the
> clinical nurse consultant involved: "We're a district nursing service. We visit people at
> home. Shut down this clinic". And I'm going, "Excuse me, but we have all this". "Nope,
> shut it down". She told the nurse involved, "No more, you go out to see patients". So, when

her supervisor came out, they asked us, "Where is the clinic?" And we go, "She told us to shut it down". Her response: "No, I didn't. You chose to. That was you". Really psychopathic stuff.

Chris faced moving goalposts from her boss, who seemed determined to push her into resigning. Her working conditions and the type of work she was allowed to do changed. She was stopped from doing the work she loved and was skilled at. In one instance, her work role changed entirely and was downgraded well below her position level and description:

> The bully would do anything to get rid of me. So, she orchestrated a way to ensure I would leave the organisation. She knew what things were important to me, and she systematically took all those things away. She stopped me from being able to do a group. She took me off the program I was working on that I had set up and loved. She changed my work hours. I was told that I wouldn't be able to work from home anymore. They stopped me from doing all the tasks I was employed to do. Instead, they said I would do administrative tasks, photocopying, and saving things to USBs.

Reflecting on her experiences, Chris saw changing the goalposts as a tactic bullies used to undermine staff and control the environment. This left staff feeling powerless and unable to flourish and achieve in their area of work:

> There was just lots of self-promoting and lots of grand plans. Nothing was ever followed through, and everything was very disorganised. Things constantly changed and shifted, "Hang on, we just changed. What was the purpose of that? I'm not really sure that there's any good reason other than you're trying to keep us all up in the air because that's easier to control people". It wasn't warm and fuzzy. It was my way or the highway.

In my case, it felt more like being a ping pong ball in a very long game between the health service and the university. I had a contract position ending, and I wanted it renewed. I took all the figures and showed that long service leave savings could cover it. That wasn't enough. The senior nurse wanted the university to pay half. So off I went to see the dean, who surprisingly agreed. Great, so I forwarded the information to the faculty business manager. I received a response that the senior nurse had never agreed (despite it being in writing) and would not commit. I went back to the dean, assuming she would still provide her promised support, and got a flat no. All that back and forward when they could have just said no in the first place. That stuff happened all the time. It was so frustrating, so wearying.

Exploiting Vulnerability

> I said: "Well, if I don't take leave, I'll run myself into the ground because that's where I'm heading". Her response: zip, zilch, zero, nothing (Jordan).

The importance of working in a supportive and mentally healthy workplace has been increasingly placed in the spotlight. Employer assistance programs, for example, provide (albeit limited) counselling for employees. Some organisations have extensive programs to support mental health and well-being. Therefore, it would seem reasonable to expect all staff, particularly managers, to respect and enact the importance of mental health and well-being. For health services, this should be a "no brainer". People are happier and more productive if they are treated well and supported. This means better outcomes for patients, students, trainers, or whomever they work with. Unfortunately, the champions' experiences demonstrate a stark contrast, especially when vulnerable. Andy, Pat, and Jordan felt unsupported at times of need, to the point of harassment, at other times negligence, or at the very least, failing the duty of care.

Andy was harassed by her manager while she was gravely ill and taking extended sick leave. The bully never inquired about her health and offered no support:

> Eventually, I got sick, and I don't know whether it was because of her, but certainly, it was while she was there. I was hospitalised for about a week. I could just have a shower and go back to bed for about four or five weeks. She would ring every week to say, "Are you coming back?" She wanted to know if I was coming back on Monday, and I go, "Well, you know, it's Wednesday now, I can't tell you. I am just having a shower and going back to bed. I will let you know on Monday".

Pat had only recently returned to work following brain surgery. Her manager had constantly been critical of her work performance. When Pat reminded her she had recently been seriously ill, instead of being supported, she was put through a series of hoops to prove her fitness for work:

> We had this meeting with the head of department, the bully, the manager of the service and me. She was telling me all the things I wasn't doing right, and I said, "For God's sake, I have been in hospital. I've had brain tumours removed". She looked at me with these wide eyes and said, "You've had brain surgery?" I said, "Look, it's not a secret". Everybody knew. Everybody in the hospital I was in contact with knew what had happened. She said, "Well, I'm going to have to go to HR and tell them because you shouldn't be driving". I said, "Says who that I can't drive?" She asked if I had approval. I said, "I haven't received anything saying I can't drive, and if my surgeon or specialist were concerned, they would have had my licence cancelled". The next minute they put me on forced leave, and I was out of work for about three weeks waiting for a letter saying I was safe to drive. Then they wanted an independent medical assessment done, and this guy said, I couldn't return to work because I couldn't get down on my knees to perform CPR. Not that that was part of my job anyway. Again, I was put on forced leave until that assessment had been done. I knew there was something wrong. I just couldn't put my finger on it. I said, "I'm not processing the information; I'm not remembering everything. I put things in place like checklists and using diaries and post-it notes, but I'm still missing stuff, and I don't know why". Then they sent me for a neuropsych assessment, and I scored pretty high on that, bearing in mind the office I worked in was an open plan and very noisy. I had asked if I could return to where I used to sit with colleagues because then I've got someone there that I can say, "How do we do this or what do we do about this now?" And she told me I couldn't do that and needed to get out of my comfort zone. This just kept going on and on.

Jordan was completely dumbfounded by her bosses at the hospital and the university's continual failure to acknowledge her vulnerability and distress. Even when she let them know she was struggling, they offered no support:

There are a couple of instances that I remember. I was talking to the senior nurse as I was taking long service leave, and she wanted to know how the staff would manage without me. How would they know what work to do? I tried to assure her that they were very capable of working without supervision. In the end, I said: "Well, if I don't take leave, I'll run myself into the ground because that's where I'm heading". Her response: zip, zilch, zero, nothing. Where was the duty of care? Where was "is there anything I can do? Do you have support? Have you gone to the employee assistance program? How bad is this?" Not a single solitary word. The research director was just as bad. I had been talking about my issues for ages. Finally, one day I'd had enough. I said to him, "Nobody has said anything to me about support. No one has asked if I am having counselling. For goodness' sake, this is a Department of Health, and you're a psychologist. What's that all about?" to this day. I do not understand how people can be so insensitive and utterly lacking in empathy. Even if they don't like me, what about the legal ramifications if I was to throw myself under a bus or smash my car into a pole or any of the things people are more likely to do when they're under extreme stress? It absolutely defied logic.

My life is unrecognisable from what it was before I went to work here. I struggle a lot with suicidal ideation and suicidal thoughts (Alex).

Increased attention to workplace bullying has strengthened interest in, and understanding of, its impact on the people targeted and the community more broadly. Workplace bullying costs the Australian economy an estimated $36 billion annually through sick leave, reduced productivity, staff turnover, legal action, and reputational damage. A figure likely to be much higher if the impact of subtle forms of bullying, often unrecognised, were included.

Economics is one factor. Undoubtedly, bullying profoundly affects all aspects of target's lives. At work, it can shatter confidence, self-esteem, enjoyment, and a sense of fulfilment. It can create fear, anxiety, and avoidant behaviour, resulting in severe isolation. No one can work effectively in a toxic environment. A deeply distressing aspect of bullying is that its influence doesn't stop at the end of the working day. Bullying potentially impacts every part of the targets' lives. Sleep disturbance, substance misuse, relationship issues, and loss of enjoyment are commonly described.

Hearing about how intensely their experiences had affected the champions was deeply disturbing. Their lives had been profoundly changed. The impact for some will likely be forever. They had all loved their jobs, and their work and career were so much a part of their lives and who they were as people. They experienced intensely personal emotions and loss of confidence and often found themselves doubting if it were real or if they were to blame. Bullying affected their health and well-being and capacity to do their job to the standard they expected of themselves. It was heartbreaking. Once again, I struggled with the thought that my experiences were nothing and had to remind myself that it wasn't a competition. I too had experiences that broke my heart.

5.1   The Love of the Job

> I love my job. I love the staff that I work with. I just hate coming and being treated like this (Sam).

One of the hardest parts for the champions was the "shattering" of their love of the job. It was for me. My work has always been so much a part of me. I work harder than I need to because I love it. I take great pride and receive so much satisfaction. When the work environment is positive, I am creative, diligent, and unstoppable. I am literally crushed when I am blocked, ignored, micromanaged, and face moving goalposts. The effect on my psyche is enormous. It slows me down from doing the job I am paid to do, the job I am good at, and the job I love. I become frustrated. If I'm doing something wrong or not doing something I should be, tell me! For goodness' sake, tell me. Don't just start treating me like I don't exist. It is so pointless. Why do these bullies so often put-up blocks for the hardest workers?

When Pat returned to work after a severe and life-threatening illness, going back to the job she loved was an important part of her recovery. She loved her job, and being back at work meant she was returning to the old her:

> When I had my leaving afternoon tea, a colleague told me how she remembered seeing me in hospital. All I was worried about was coming back to work. In a way, it was what got me through. In a couple of months, I can go back to work. It was a bit like, well, if I get back to work, that means I'm going to be back to where I was before I got sick.

Terry and Sam found the weight of bullying so much heavier because their work was so important in their lives and for their sense of self:

Terry: I have intense feelings of unfairness. It was distressing in everything I did because my work is so important to me, so being under pressure at work really derails my focus in life. It detaches me from the thing that usually gives me so much pleasure.

Sam: I love my job. I love the staff that I work with. I just hate coming and being treated like this.

5.2   Dreading Work

> I would cry all the way from our house, about an hour to where I worked, and it would be like, "What am I going to be in for when I get in today? (Pat)".

From loving their jobs, some champions now found themselves in sheer dread about going to work. Pat and Andy were constantly on edge about what they may face from the bully:

Pat: I'd get up of a morning and cry and sob and say to my partner, "Do I have to go to work today?" He'd say, "Yeah, you've got to go in". I'd say, "But I don't want to go in". He'd say, "You've got to go". I would cry all the way from our house, about an hour to where I worked, and it would be like, "What am I going to be in for when I get in today?"

Andy: I would feel a sense of dread. I often had that sense of God, what next? Do I have to go today? There's always the chance not to go today. Sometimes I might be thinking thank God she's got lots of meetings today. She is not going to be there. It's going to be okay.

For Jordan, dreading work was not confined to being at the office or even during conventional working hours. She could receive unwelcome and imposing communications anywhere at any time:

> The sense of dread was constant. It wasn't just not wanting to go to work. I did so much of my work and communication via email, so I could never be sure what would happen next. There was always a chance I would get an email asking me where I was and what I was doing. Or the boss would let me know she wasn't happy with something in her surly authoritarian tone. Even in my own home or on the other side of the world, a great day could be completely thrown into chaos. An email could arrive with unreasonable demands or inappropriate and passive-aggressive criticism. It was there 24 hours a day, at least potentially. It's bloody hard when you can't escape it.

Shannon's dread about going to work had become so overwhelming she likened it to her experiences of depression:

> I fear going back to work on Thursday. I had Monday off sick. Sick of work, maybe. And so, I worked Friday, and then I won't work again until Thursday. There'll be a plethora of information I don't get, and I'll be on the back foot again. I've probably gone back about 10 feet. I have suffered depression. I had post-natal depression, and I can only align it with that by saying, vocationally, I feel at the bottom of a deep dark hole. There's no ladder, and there's no way out. But I can't see anyone giving me a leg up here. It's a terrible feeling. It's a really terrible feeling.

5.3   Loss of Self-Confidence and Self-Doubt

> I constantly doubted myself. Am I seeing this? Is this happening? These people are so good at keeping you guessing and ripping the rug out from under you (Chris).

Because the bullying was persistent and often insidious, champions found their self-image and self-confidence badly damaged. They often doubted themselves and wondered if the problem was imagined or if the behaviours were their fault. This was gradual for me. Initially, I thought I was just unlucky. "She's a bitch". I didn't take it on board and probably not the next time either. When it kept happening, from good boss to bad boss, good boss suddenly becomes bad boss; I started thinking, is this about me? Is it something I do? I certainly didn't intend it to be. All I've ever wanted is to do a good job.

For Shannon, her first experience of bullying came as a complete shock. It affected her confidence, and she became isolated from her colleagues:

The bullying just shut me down. I lost all of my confidence. I really, really felt isolated. Because I'd been removed from my team. Even though I'd self-removed because I felt I had to, all the consequences were for me.

For Rory, Chris, and Sam, bullying created self-doubt and left them questioning whether they were somehow responsible for what they were experiencing:

Rory: I still have these moments of "maybe they're right?" Maybe this was all my fault. This is my personality, and maybe I am a terrible person who deserved this. I still have all these thoughts, and it's hard when you've had such awful things said about you.

Chris: I constantly doubted myself. Am I seeing this? Is this happening? These people are so good at keeping you guessing and ripping the rug out from under you.

Sam: I've reflected on all sorts of things about the part I play. Do I behave in a different way? Do I become defensive? That's when you go through that reflection. Is this really happening? Is it just me? Is it in my head?

As an experienced psychologist, Lee became very knowledgeable about bullying from her own experiences, observations, training, and research. Despite her knowledge and expertise, self-doubt still crept in, and she constantly reflected on her own behaviour and actions:

You can know it intellectually, and you can see it, and you can read, and I've probably read 50 books on bullying. At the university we had to have anti-bullying training every single year. I've helped people and supported people who were being bullied. Yet, when you're in the middle of it, you can – be a mental health professional for 25 years, I still sit there and go, "What the fuck was I doing there? What was I thinking?" You doubt yourself. You start to think, "Am I difficult, am I negative?" Luckily, I'm still in close contact with the 12 people who did leave, "Oh, actually, no, they're telling me I'm right". I'm sitting back and thinking, or I'm now listening to the taped conversation of the general meeting going, "No, I was not rude, I did not have tone, I wasn't eating. How on earth did you say I'm being negative about something?"

Self-doubt became persistent and overwhelming for Taylor. She needed support to appreciate the most important things in her life and better understand the motives of the bullies:

I get really exhausted from the anxiety of trying so hard. I get really down on myself. Maybe they're right, and I'm wrong. If you have been deemed as "insane" and been submerged, by others, in all the negative connotations that people with "severe and enduring" mental health issues have loaded upon them. If you have experienced what it feels like to doubt your own mind, you can quickly and frequently jump to "maybe you are wrong, and they are right". I'm lucky, I have a loving, lovely partner and wonderful children and grandchildren. So, when it's all getting too much for me, my partner helps me get perspective by asking, "If you were on your death bed, what would you think was most important?" But that's the purpose of bullying. It's to break you. It's to make you lose confidence. It's to make you look stupid, inept, and "mad" in a negative sense of the word.

From self-doubt and loss of confidence, Pat constantly questioned her ability to do her job. She became so fearful of making mistakes she considered leaving as an escape from the stress and tension of the job:

> I was always guessing whether I was doing things correctly or doing a good enough job. You were waiting for someone to tap you on the shoulder and say, "You didn't do this, or you didn't do that". You make mistakes because you're learning, and they were all experts. I just felt that I didn't want to learn anything. I didn't want to know. I just wanted to get out of there, and that's what I focused on. I remember saying to someone that if I could find a job in a bookshop or selling flowers, I'd be happy because this is just not worth the grief, the self-doubt, and the sleepless nights.

Pat questioned her skills and knowledge so deeply that she needed reassurance from a colleague that her ability was not the problem. Reassurance was not enough to overcome her negative feelings towards herself:

> It made me question my skills as a health professional. It was only a friend of mine from school who is also a health professional who said to me, "Look, you've still got those skills, don't let her beat you down". But it's really hard to try and be upbeat and positive when every day you're facing this.

The impact of two experiences of extreme bullying left Rory feeling totally devastated. Her confidence was so battered that she seriously considered leaving medicine entirely:

> I had these two horrible experiences and didn't really feel that I had any confidence in my abilities. So, I didn't really want to go through that again. I was so angry at the processes and the culture, and the lack of support, and I guess I didn't know if I could go back to that.

5.4 Fear

> I go to work, and I want to throw up, and I hide in my office. I am scared, and I don't acknowledge it anymore (Terry).

Faced with severe bullying or the threat of it, day after day, left some champions becoming so fearful they experienced physical or psychological symptoms and sometimes both:

Alex: I was vomiting during my shift, I was having trouble controlling my bladder, I was having dizziness, nausea, and the headaches I was experiencing were extreme.

Terry's fear of being ignored by colleagues resulted in avoidance:

> I have fear avoidance behaviour. When I go to the hospital, I go straight into my office, lock the door behind me, and then sneak out again, hoping I won't meet anyone. Sometimes I felt ready to throw up. I didn't want to meet people in the corridor because I know people I say hello to will walk past me and ignore me. So, I am flat-out afraid of going there. When people pass me and ignore me, it kills me. It really does. I'm avoiding this place, and I'm not happy. In my relationship with the world, I am denied something when people ignore

me. And it gets to me to the extent that I'm ready to just go home, cry, and never come back to that workplace.

Terry had been fearful for so long. It was so ingrained that he had become less aware of it and saw it as a normal part of the environment:

I'm so used to it that I don't know how stressful it is, and that's why I struggle to put into words that I actually go to work, and I'm scared. I go to work, and I want to throw up, and I hide in my office. I am scared, and I don't acknowledge it anymore.

Sam often found herself fearful in meetings. She worried that the information she needed had been deliberately withheld and she was at risk of being shown up as unprepared or lacking in front of colleagues:

It makes it very hard because you're missing pieces of the puzzle. And when you still need pieces of the puzzle, you can't give the completed piece to the people you work with. I can go into meetings thinking I know what I am talking about, but it's possible I am missing important bits. I sometimes get really anxious if I know I'm going to be in the same room as her. How does it affect my work? Without the information, it is very hard to do my job, especially if I have problems with my managers. Anybody, if they can see a split, they will make it wider.

The fear Chris experienced became so strong she didn't feel safe being alone with the bully:

I didn't even feel safe meeting with her one-on-one. If I had to meet with her, I asked for the door to be left open because she'd yelled at me before. My biggest concern was that if I were left alone with her, she would say I threatened her. Because she did, she made out that I yelled at her, that I'd done all these things I hadn't done.

Taylor found herself debilitated by fear. She did her job as best she could, given the barriers she faced. Reflecting on her experiences, she considered the bullies were creating an environment of fear as an intentional strategy to keep targets under control:

You become fearful. And that's why they do it, to intimidate you to the point where you won't make waves. You become fearful that each time you put in a complaint or ask for something on behalf of somebody else, it will mount up. The way bullies treat you gets worse and worse. It is frightening. I still did my job, but I could have done a better job with less damage to me and better outcomes for all if I had felt safe to do it.

5.5   Why Can't I Cope?

I should be able to cope with this. I should be able to push through. I should be able to do this (Andy).

Andy and Jordan asked themselves this question often. They felt they had failed because they were so strongly affected. They constantly questioned their own reactions and admonished themselves for spending so much time and energy on the people responsible for the bullying and toxicity:

Andy: I just felt like I'd failed because I should be able to cope. That was the key for me. I should be able to cope with this. I should be able to push through. It created a sense of stress because I didn't know how to cope with that. I didn't know how to resolve it.

Jordan: The fact I let it get to me so much played heavily on me at times. I kept thinking about all the great things I had in my life and why I didn't focus more on them. Sometimes it made me feel worse than the bullying itself. There's a lot of stuff around that says don't let people get to you. They're not worth it. Focus on the good stuff, all of that. No argument, but it's just not that easy. Sometimes it made me feel worse that not only was I being bullied, but I wasn't even responding to it the way it should be.

5.6   Losing Friends and Colleagues

> When your colleagues, those you look up to, whom you have fought beside for reform, judge you, usurp you, undermine you, bully you or intimidate you, it is harder. (Taylor).

The loss of collegiate relationships and friendships was one of the most challenging impacts of bullying on the champions. I saw a quote somewhere that you don't lose friends; you lose undercover haters. It amused me. I wouldn't go that far. I certainly lost people I had believed to be my friends, which was undoubtedly the hardest part of the bullying ordeal. It wasn't even so much that I lost them, although sometimes I was very sad about that. It was more that I had spent so much of my time, trust, and faith and had enjoyed the company of people who would sell me down the river in a heartbeat. One of the saddest was a work colleague I became very close to. She had some personal issues in her life, and she trusted me as the one person to confide in. I remember how honoured I felt. The relationship started to cool off when she moved into a higher position within the school. She humiliated me in front of a staff member on one occasion. Even though we sorted through that, things were never the same. In hindsight, she must have known the powers that be in the school wanted me gone. I know many people would do the same thing, under those circumstances, preserve their own job and career. Still, it did surprise me about her because this wasn't just an ordinary friendship. What would I have done in that situation? I honestly don't think I could be complicit with anyone being treated that way. I keep asking myself, how do health professionals treat each other so badly?

Most champions had also lost friends and colleagues because of bullying. Pat and Shannon found this particularly hard because they had enjoyed an active social life and close relationships through work:

Pat: One of my colleagues got married, and I went to her wedding. Another one had a baby, and I'd made a blanket for the baby. We've had lunches together and caught up outside of work. I've gone over to people's homes for meals, and they've come here for meals. So that was really, really devastating at the time.

Shannon: My work was my social life. Four of us were single mums, and we would socialise together, and that slowly started to drift off. I was so upset, I probably went on about it too much. And they probably didn't want to hear about it. I don't know. And even though these people had supported me during the bullying incident, no one followed up after I went on leave.

For Jordan losing friendships was the most challenging part of her bullying experiences. She talked of two relationships that had been destroyed through bullying. Even several years later, she still felt immense sadness at the loss:

I had a very close colleague and friend for years. He became an advisor and confidant, and I trusted him implicitly, which was rare for me. I also considered him a good friend. The organisation he worked for was a partner in the centre I was running. His boss was a bully and gave me a really hard time over the years. I have no doubt that my trusted colleague did not support me. I don't know whether he directly contributed to the passive bullying, although sadly, I suspect he did. When I was leaving, I asked him to speak at my farewell. I have regretted that ever since because events immediately before and after showed me that he didn't mean a word he said. He was glad to see me go. I barely heard from him after I left. He actually criticised me because my silence towards his bully boss made people uncomfortable. I hadn't lost him. He had never really been a friend or even a decent colleague. The fact he was so disingenuous and lacking real substance. It was very, very hurtful.

Another lost friendship upset me greatly. I believed we were friends and definitely respected colleagues. She head hunted me for the job. When she left, our relationship changed dramatically. I could only conclude that I was no longer useful to her. We worked on projects, publications, and grant applications. I did most of the work but included her, not because she was a friend but because she was a colleague, and that was how I rolled. What really upset me was how she treated me after that. We sat on a management committee together, and she disagreed with pretty much everything I said. She would make her points in a blunt and hostile manner. I can be direct, but I'm not rude. She was rude and disrespectful. Her judgement was so clouded by the fact that she didn't like me anymore. I was no longer useful to her (Jordan).

Jordan concluded from her experiences that many colleagues in the university environment were only collegial when there was something in it for them. They were quick to turn away when this was no longer the case:

Colleagues! Being health professionals didn't make them immune from being selfish and opportunistic. One place I worked at stands out. I invested a lot of my time mentoring colleagues, helping them get publications and building their track record. I was incredibly generous with authorship. Several staff achieved promotions which were at least supported by my contribution. When I took on a new role, I didn't have as much time for that, and thought they could step up on their own. I was simply no longer useful to them. Only one or two were openly hostile. The others more or less ignored me. Sadly, what I had done and achieved apparently meant nothing when I left. Of the many people I had worked closely with, only two had anything nice to say to me or acknowledged my contribution. Others did not even bother to say goodbye. It was like I had never been there. I don't understand how people with that attitude can walk into a classroom and talk to students about empathy or person-centred care. It's an absolute joke.

Lee described losing both friends and colleagues because of the bullying and the part she played in removing the bully:

> I do think some were damaged. There were people who didn't really bond with the CEO but just looked at where their bread-and-butter lay and went, "I will put my head down and look after myself" and didn't stand up when she did terrible things to other people. Even though they did nothing personally to me, it is really hard to respect them. There are also some people who, when we were going through the worst of it, thought I was stronger than that. Some people were almost like, "I know she wasn't great, but did you really have to rock the boat?" Some people that left, I think in other circumstances we would have remained friends, but they just wanted to put the place behind them.

The effect of the bullying on Taylor's relationship with colleagues only hit her when she was leaving the organisation. No one other than her own team attended her farewell. She was both surprised and extremely hurt:

> I was there for four years. I thought I had good relationships with some of the nurses and, ridiculously, desired to. I wanted to be part of that service. I'd been to a lot of farewells for staff, and 30, 60 people would attend. When I was leaving, only my team went. None of the other staff would go. So that told me that I never belonged there. They never saw me as one of them. They only ever saw me as a hindrance at best and the enemy at worst. I was hurt and disappointed. I was also embarrassed. Embarrassed that I'd ever thought there was anything more there. I do think that with clinical staff for their safety and well-being, they felt that they couldn't be seen as an ally of mine. The few that were got hell from the bullies.

Taylor also talked about the impact of bullying on collegiate relationships in her broader professional community. One relationship was damaged after she had expressed a genuine and honest opinion that was not well received:

> I lost somebody I wouldn't consider a close friend but a very strong ally and a peer. I challenged peer workers at a conference. We should have proven ourselves by that time to have been really valuable, irreplaceable, and highly regarded. I was fully aware of the stigma and discrimination we experience at the hand of many clinical staff. However, we should each be asking ourselves what are we doing to not make the need for our positions obvious? We can't just play the blame game all the time. And this person really turned against me and tried to set people against me for doing that. I acknowledged how hard it was and the bullying and intimidation we got from health professionals. But we still always have to look at our responsibility in things and try and improve the situation and not play the victim game all the time. So, when this person's voice and other advocates' voices were undermining me, it was really difficult for me.

Lack of support and collegiality from peers was particularly hurtful for Taylor. She was angry about the impact on the broader professional environment and the barriers that limited the potential achievements of organisations and movements:

> You do want to be accepted, appreciated and respected by your peers. You're always second-guessing yourself anyway, whether what you're saying is right. When your colleagues, those you look up to, whom you have fought beside for reform, judge you, usurp you, undermine you, bully you or intimidate you, it is harder. You expect your peers to be on your side, the side of reform and humane treatment. If they turn against you, you feel very judged, lonely, and much more insecure about yourself and the value you bring. It's not just

frustrating. It breaks my heart. The person who has usurped my career at several stages, if they had taken me under their wing and had taught me what they knew and had worked with me, because they have different strengths to what I have. Together, what we could have achieved. I get really angry and broken-hearted about it. What right did they have to stop us from achieving all we could by working together for our community? How dare they stop us from achieving that? I find that unconscionable. Our movement, our community, I really believe we would have been a lot further along if we had worked collegially together. From where we've started, the voice of lived experience is much more heard than it used to be. We pushed that a lot, but we were doing it separately. Together, we could have done so much more. It's appalling and unconscionable. An orchestra is made up of many different instruments to make beautiful music.

Sam had been protected from the hurt of losing friends because she quite intentionally kept a clear separation between her work and personal life:

> I keep work very separate. There are people I consider very important in my life that I work with but don't socialise with, that I know would have my back in a minute, like my boss. I know what they think of me. But I don't socialise with them. Once every two years, we go out. I try and keep the two separate, which may be helpful, or maybe it's not.

Pat found herself excluded by most colleagues. What she heard from one person suggested the fear of becoming the next victim by association was probably why her workmates drew away from her:

> I had colleagues I'd worked with for 12 years who wouldn't sit with me at lunchtime because they didn't want to be the next person targeted by this manager. There was one girl, and we used to get on really, really well. We'd have coffee on days off. She would ignore me. It was just like I wasn't there. I'd walk past and say hello, and she wouldn't even acknowledge me, really? I thought, what's going on? Have they been told not to sit with me? One of them said, "It's not that I don't want to talk to you. I don't want to be seen talking to you" because the manager had already said some things to her.

Similarly, Jesse saw her exclusion by colleagues as a conscious decision to side with the bully and be active supporters of his behaviour:

> The other managers at my level started to treat me differently. There was no support there. There was a fair bit of negativity, and I felt very mobbed by it. People felt they had a blessing to be mean. They really were on his side, and I didn't get any support from them at all. I supervised one of the ladies' Masters, and we were quite close. I'd done my PhD with a couple of them. So, I would've felt we had a fairly good relationship.

Responses from colleagues created a dilemma for Andy and Chris. While they understood the need for self-preservation, it was still hurtful to be abandoned by colleagues:

Andy: I was probably the first one affected by that manager, although later on, they all got to see what she was like. Quite a number resigned on their own. It's like, I'm telling you the facts, and I'm not making this shit up. I understand self-preservation, I do get that because you don't want it to rain down on you, but I'd worked with them a lot longer than they'd worked with her. So, I wouldn't go as strong as betrayed, just very disappointed. I do get it, but I also don't. It's very hard. It's an insular little group, particularly at the management level. I think they didn't want to say anything too much, so they didn't become the next target. I understand that, but it is hurtful. It's disappointing.

Chris: I had two responses. One was to feel really annoyed that I had amazing relationships with so many of the team. It was hard to think that people could not even check in. What do we all stand for? We're mental health nurses, and we can't even look after each other, I'd told management about this person bullying other people. I tried to have other people's backs. Only three reached out to say, "We've got no idea what happened, but we just wanted you to know that we really enjoyed working with you". Everyone else - you could hear a pin drop. The other part of me was thinking much more black and white. I didn't reach out to any of them because I didn't want them to have the same experience. I knew that if I had gone to them with everything that had happened, some would have had targets on their back. I didn't want to make other people's lives difficult. Because I'd had this experience of going to management, and management just telling me, oh, we think you're lying about it all. Go away. It would have had to be a number of them all saying the same thing for management to do anything about this situation. So, it was weird. On the one hand, I was annoyed, disappointed, and hurt. And on the other hand, I was like, yeah, I get it.

5.7   With Me Always

> It's like a cancer. It really just envelopes everything. For me, it did. It just enveloped everything (Shannon).

The bullying permeated all aspects of the champions' lives. Even away from work, the feelings and emotions the bullying created remained with them and made other aspects of their lives more difficult. Despite making a conscious effort to look after herself and do things she enjoyed, Chris found maintaining her previous active lifestyle so much harder:

> I still prioritised self-care. I don't drink alcohol or take drugs. I tried to do all the right things, catching up with friends, but everything was much harder and much more of an effort. I had to really try to make sure I wasn't always talking about this thing, even though it felt like it was always on my mind. It was horrible. And I still think it took me at least a year of healing.

Pat, Andy, Rory, and Shannon also found it very challenging to do things they enjoyed, as the bullying weighed heavily and went with them everywhere:

Pat: I didn't enjoy weekends because it was in the back of my mind. I hated Sundays because tomorrow is Monday, and you've got another 5 days of work. So, I hated Sundays. We'd go out in the boat, and I didn't enjoy it at all, whereas before, I loved going out in the boat on the weekend or spending time with family.

Andy: You're thinking ahead all the time. I would be in the shower, I would be trying to sleep or wake up thinking about things to do at work, and then I would start to think about, oh my god, that person. What is going to happen tomorrow? What are goalposts going to change?

Rory: I really struggled. Certainly, my sleep was affected, and my mood was affected. I was living with housemates, so at least I'd come home and interact with them, but I definitely was doing fewer social activities. When I first moved there, I was doing heaps of outdoor activities. I was still trying. It just wasn't the same. I was doing it to try to clear my head rather than anything else. So, it wasn't as enjoyable. I wasn't communicating with any of my friends or family back home either.

Shannon: It's like a cancer. It really just envelopes everything. For me, it did. It just enveloped everything. And I think had I had a partner, they probably would have left me. But I didn't, luckily. I had a dog.

I can absolutely relate. For me, the effect of bullying on weekends and evenings was worse than working hours, with more time and fewer distractions. At work, I had focus. I had a diversion. At home, I often continued working because I didn't have the motivation or energy to do anything else. I would think to myself, you've got to go out this weekend. You've got to do something, but I was just so exhausted. Even cleaning up the house and doing the washing sometimes felt just too hard. I'm so lucky I had a supportive partner. I don't know what I would've done. I don't know how I would've managed. To be honest, I don't know if I'd still be here.

For Alex, the effects of bullying were so pervasive she believed she had lost her independence and become a burden to her family:

It's horrific every single day, and I'm a burden to my family. My son lives with us now, and he and my husband take care of me and do everything. I can't do things that I used to be able to do, and it is devastating. I was always a very independent person, and to have every bit of your identity and independence stripped from you, you have no dignity anymore.

After two episodes of life-threatening illness, Pat felt shattered and exhausted by the relentless bullying:

I kept saying to my mum and my partner, why did I fight so hard to get through the cancer and the treatment if this is what I'm now faced with? I should have just given up.

5.8   Sleep

It made me tired. It made me anxious. I haven't slept since July because you've always not done enough (Lee).

We are all very conscious of how vital sleep is for our health and well-being, especially when dealing with the stress of constant bullying. Knowing that does not make it easy to deal with, and sleep was an issue for nearly all champions. It certainly was for me. Constant rumination made restful sleep almost impossible. Lack of sleep had a flow on effect to other aspects of the champions' lives:

Chris: I had poor sleep, I'd cry a lot, and my self-esteem and self-confidence plummeted. Lots of worrying thoughts and rumination. Even though I knew what all this was and why I was experiencing what I was experiencing, it was still hard to try and manage it.

Lee: It made me tired. It made me anxious. I haven't slept since July because you've always not done enough.

Taylor: I didn't sleep much. In those years, I was operating on around three and a half to four hours of broken sleep a night.

Ruminating about bullying made sleep particularly difficult for Sam:

> If it is playing on my mind, sometimes I'll be angry, and I don't sleep, and I will find myself thinking about an email she's written or something like that. And in my head, going over how I am going to address it.

For Terry, the impact of the bullying was so profound it led to nightmares:

> I sometimes have nightmares about it because I don't have any control. So, I feel like there are a lot of demands on me, but I don't have control over how to get out of it.

Pat and Lee talked about how the lack of sleep and tiredness affected their performance at work:

Pat: I didn't sleep at all. I'd go to bed, and it felt like my brain was spinning. There were a couple of times when I was at work and was just so tired. If I went out on a home visit, I'd pull over near a park and have a nanna nap.

Lee: Every day, I was a hundred emails behind, and it would just get worse every single day; 50 phone calls behind. Like, it was just uncatch-up-able. So, the guilt and the worry and the stuff doing lots of unpaid overtime, no sleep, stress, that sort of stuff, the impact is severe.

Jordan found the constant inability to sleep so debilitating that she resorted to medication as a strategy:

> I usually got to sleep okay. But I would wake up an hour or two later with a real rush of adrenaline, pure anxiety. I was wide awake and alert, ready to fight off goodness knows what. Sometimes I would take medication to help me sleep, and sometimes a bit more. I hated doing it, and it wasn't just because I was so tired. I couldn't stand lying there awake hour after hour, questioning why this was happening to me and wondering what I could do to stop it. When I went to bed, I often told myself: "Tonight, you won't take anything". Then I'd wake up with that horrible feeling of anxiety and all those thoughts going through my head about what was happening to me. I just couldn't stand it, so I took sleepers. I hated myself for it sometimes.

5.9   Alcohol

> I knew I was drinking too much, and that was one more thing to worry about and feel bad
> about (Jordan).

While most champions didn't drink or did so in moderation only, self-medication
through alcohol became a coping strategy for Shannon and Jordan:

Shannon: I drank far too much as a coping mechanism. I really, really felt iso-
            lated. The longer that went on, the worse it became because it created
            this whirlwind. And it just kept on re-presenting itself. If I were to see
            someone, I'd feel awkward, and I'd be socially inept.

Jordan: I drank far more than I should have. I would get home from another
            crappy day and think to myself I'll have a drink, just one. Unfortunately,
            it wasn't very often only one drink. Of course, I worried about that. I
            knew I was drinking too much, and that was one more thing to worry
            about and feel bad about.

5.10   Driven to the Edge

> I didn't feel that I would be able to stop feeling as awful as I did ... I attempted suicide and
> was admitted to the hospital after I was found the next day (Rory).

Some champions found themselves much more easily frustrated and less tolerant, which often impacted their relationships with family and intimate partners:

Lee: I still remember being – not now, but at the time – just so cross and frus-
            trated at simple things

Sam: Some days, I do take it out on the family. It's hard to separate the job and
            living with the family's stresses and needs because, maybe partially of my
            own creation, I have a relatively needy family.

Andy: Hugely, hugely. The girls and my partner are sick to death of me complain-
            ing about it. "Get another job, get another job". Well, of course, that's
            easier said than done.

Terry: It actually crops up in my intimate relationships when someone says the
            opposite of what the bully will say. I get this reaction because I've inter-
            nalised some of the bullies' ideas about me. It doesn't come up naturally,
            but it's triggered in that space.

Pat: I wasn't sleeping, I wasn't eating, I was crying every morning. I didn't
            want to go to work. My partner was getting angry with me because I wasn't
            eating and sleeping, and I was crying. He was trying to support me, but he
            didn't understand the process.

Alex's situation was particularly delicate because her partner had encouraged her
to work in the field where the bullying occurred:

> It's been hard for my partner. He feels guilty, and he feels like he is to blame for this because
> he introduced me to the Ambulance Service.

Jordan's behaviour at home became so much of a problem it almost ended her relationship:

> Looking back, my fuse was getting shorter and shorter. I knew it was about work. I knew it was a problem. I didn't know how much. Sometimes I would be so absorbed by my frustration and anger that I couldn't see what I was doing and what effect it was having. My partner bore the brunt of it. I didn't want my staff entangled, so I put on a brave face there. At home, it didn't take much, and I would overreact. I was hypersensitive. My partner was so patient. Eventually, it got to breaking point. He was on the brink of leaving, and I was thinking, "Just go". Then at the 11th hour, I thought, "What the bloody hell are you doing here?" Is your crappy job really worth your relationship? We talked. I had an event I was involved in organising, so I asked, "Can you stay with me until that is over? After that, if things get bad again, you just say the word, and I will leave my job". It was the shock to the system I needed. I knew then that whatever happened at work, I wouldn't let it end my relationship. It wasn't worth that.

The impact of bullying on Alex was horrendous, far-reaching, long-lasting, and life-threatening:

> I cannot sleep … I'm on seven different medications right now. I have severe PTSD and major depressive disorder and chronic pain syndrome. So, my sleep is awful. I had episodes where things would happen that I didn't remember. There were times I confronted my son, believing he had taken my debit card and gone shopping, and I'd actually gone on shopping trips that I didn't remember. I can't drive anymore because of that. My psychiatrist says that it's called dissociating. By the time I left work, I ended up with a hiatus hernia that had to be repaired. My doctor told them that my medical condition was life-threatening and came from the distress levels I was trying to cope with. I've become quite agoraphobic. They've done such intrusive surveillance on me that I don't feel safe leaving my house anymore. So, my life is unrecognisable from what it was before I went to work here. I struggle a lot with suicidal thoughts. Understanding everything you feel and trying to navigate those emotions becomes overwhelming.

Rory's reaction to the very real possibility of being forced to leave a job she loved because of bullying was so strong she didn't want to continue living and attempted to end her life:

> It made me really suicidal again because I thought I'd been happy here. I wanted to stay. Things were going okay, and then I had people telling me I was an awful person, they don't want me here, and I'm going to have to leave again. I'm going to have to go somewhere else and try to start afresh. I had had enough. I was devastated. I didn't want to start somewhere new. I didn't feel I would be able to stop feeling as awful as I did. I attempted suicide and was admitted to the hospital after I was found the next day. I spent several days in ICU and was transferred to my home state for ongoing inpatient psychiatric care.

Lee had two colleagues whose health and well-being were profoundly affected by bullying:

> These other two women were severely affected. One of them had a history of self-harm. She ended up self-harming when she hadn't for 10 years. The other one was off for 6 or 8 weeks at different times over this period, and they literally bullied her out of the place.

How I Responded

When you've been traumatised in the past, if you're not feeling heard, not being supported … It's really hard for those self-help strategies to have any useful degree of impact
(Taylor).

We know the impact of bullying can be profound and potentially life-threatening.
We know it affects the targets' capacity to do their job and can destroy their love of
the work. We know it doesn't stop at the end of the day and can permeate all aspects
of the targets' lives. So how do we deal with it? Can we stop it, or how it affects us?
Where do we start?

A quick internet search for "how to deal with workplace bullying?" reveals a
plethora of resources. It is positive to see so much attention given to workplace bullying. However, reading these documents, I was disappointed that many suggestions
were unhelpful and potentially damaging. Unfortunately, they fell way short of
demonstrating an understanding of the complexity and power dynamics of workplace bullying, particularly the more subtle forms. A quick summary of the main
suggestions includes:

- Keep accurate and detailed records of bullying experiences.
- Refer to the workplace bullying policy for information about processes to follow.
- Discuss behaviour with the bully and ask them to stop (without accusations of
  bullying).
- Advise your manager (or their manager if your manager is the bully) or human
  resources.
- Consult with unions.
- Register a complaint with the Fair Work Commission.
- Resign.
- Don't take it personally. It's about the bully.
- "Stay calm and rise above".
- Seek legal advice.

© The Author(s), under exclusive license to Springer Nature
Switzerland AG 2024
B. Happell, *Sickness in Health: Bullying in Nursing and other Health
Professions*, https://doi.org/10.1007/978-3-031-49336-2_6

Some suggested strategies are definitely worth considering. Some are downright offensive. "Stay calm and rise above", and "don't take it personally. It's about the bully". These statements, however well intended, do not reflect how profoundly bullying affects people in all aspects of their lives. The experiences of the champions presented in this book provide voice to what many of us know only too well. This is not a schoolyard spat. It's not a matter of rising above. It's challenging not to take things personally when the bullies have the power to attack your self-worth and make it difficult, if not impossible, to do your job effectively. These sentiments come very close to blaming the victim. I see statements like "you're only bullied if you allow yourself to be" all too often, even on anti-bullying media. The responsibility for bullying lies with the bully and that must never be lost sight of. Don't take it personally should be replaced with "know it's not your fault".

All these suggestions were tried by at least one champion. In most cases, they weren't effective and sadly often made a bad situation worse. This chapter describes how champions attempted to deal with bullying. Some are still ongoing. Most champions tried to address the underlying issues. Some ultimately left the workplace, while others are still working with the bully and continuing their attempts to reach a resolution.

6.1   Subtle Bullying Is Hard to Prove

It's just that grain of sand in your shoe. One grain is nothing, but then you add the next one and the next one and the next one, and then you get a blister (Andy).

In Bully Tactics, the champions described subtle forms of bullying as the most common. Their efforts to deal with situations were hampered by the often-intangible nature of events. Examples of bullying were constant and cumulative rather than clear and specific, as Terry, Andy, and Jordan spoke of:

Terry: Most of the stuff is subliminal, and this is the hard part. How do you prove exclusion when you are not included?

Andy: It's hard to say, "Look, she's being so mean to me". But I am in the lab that is the busiest all the time. It sounds so pathetic, and it's just that grain of sand in your shoe. One grain is nothing, but then you add the next one and the next one and the next one, and then you get a blister. "Okay, so I didn't hear about that", another grain. "You're going to put me on call before my day off? It doesn't happen to anybody else. Okay". Another grain of sand. How will I say she's making me work harder than everyone else? She's not giving me information. How can I validate this because it's so subtle? If you didn't know, you wouldn't see it.

Jordan: It's tough to deal with that subtle bullying. What is it that you can complain about? So, your emails aren't answered, and you're not given the information you need. I can't imagine HR would give that any oxygen. If they did, "Oh goodness me, I'm sorry I've been so busy". Anyone who goes to those lengths to subtly bully you will not come around and say, "oh gosh, you caught me. I promise never to do it again". More likely, they will dish it right back to you in spades. Yelling and screaming and abusive emails, I'll take it any day. At least it gives something concrete to work with.

Shannon and Pat were asked to provide evidence when they reported the behaviour or confronted the bully. However, the subtle nature of the bullying made it really hard to do this on the spot:

Shannon: When I called out bullying the last time, I was told I needed evidence to support my case. That was the difficulty. There was very little evidence. Things like not being included. Not having all the facts and the information. So, we were told to address it when it happened and to forward an email to the manager every time. And it just fell on deaf ears because it seemed like we were being very petty. But when it's over and over and over again. As clinicians, we started to second-guess our skills. It's damaging. I can see how it wears people down.

Pat: I remember going into her office and saying, "Do you want me on this team or not?" And she said, "I can't believe that you asked that question", and I said, "I feel that you are nit-picking everything that I do". She said, "give me an example", and I couldn't, off the top of my head. When I walked out, I thought, oh, I should have said this, this, this, and this, but at the time just couldn't think.

6.2   Self-protection

When the complaint was made about my public expression of opinion, the senior managers weren't letting it go. I had the union involved, who were really supportive, and the university had HR. The tone of communication was threatening, and I was caught in a bind. I believe strongly in freedom of speech. Part of me wanted to stand on the moral high ground, defend the principles, and refuse to apologise. Sadly, I was very fragile after a long path of bullying. I had been offered another job and was preparing to leave. I wanted to go on my time frame, not theirs. Ultimately, I agreed to apologise, so they had no justification for sacking me. I don't know how carefully she read the apology. It was one of those "I did not intend to cause any offence, and I apologise for any offence caused", which, when you read it carefully, means there is really no apology at all other than perhaps for her fragile or overinflated ego. I "gave in" because I had to look after myself. I regretted it for a long time because I had let down my principles.

Champions developed strategies to protect themselves and to cope as best they could. These included documenting, trying to adapt, and self-care:

Documenting

> I was very grateful I had put so much in writing. If that had just been a conversation, I have no doubt she would've denied … that I had ever mentioned my stress levels (Jordan).

I am a great believer in documentation. Email is wonderful for keeping track of bullies and their lies, deceit, and broken promises. I've always kept emails. I can't tell you how often one of my bullies would say, "I never said that. I never promised that", and out would come the email. "Oh yes, you did!" With one bully, I would print the email, highlight the relevant section, and put it in her pigeonhole. I'd take a more subtle approach now. At least I didn't do it in meetings and expose her to embarrassment like she did with me.

Having been bullied before, Chris learned the value of documentation. She was very careful to make sure everything was in writing in case she needed to provide evidence at any point:

> From very early on, I knew I had to protect myself and make sure everything was in writing. If you have a verbal meeting, you need to follow it up with an email to get confirmation. I've seen this before. I know what's going on here and knew from the get-go about having everything documented, on this day, at this time, to be really, very thorough.

Jordan had often used documentation and her email trail as evidence when bullies tried to twist or deny a version of events:

> After a very distressing meeting with the dean, I sent her an email outlining my concerns about how the meeting had progressed. I reminded her I was very stressed, with no support or advice offered. She had the gall to reply that she was not aware of this. So out came the emails and a formal letter I had written. I highlighted the parts where I had months before I let her know the impact it was having on me. Her reply? No acknowledgement of that, no apology. I was very grateful I had put so much in writing. If that had just been a conversation, I have no doubt she would've denied to the end of the earth that I had ever mentioned my stress levels to her.

While Shannon was working at home during COVID-19, she planned to take advantage of electronic communication as a record of bullying behaviour she could produce as evidence if required in the future:

> I will put everything in writing now on the Teams App. It's true time. I posted the other day, "I don't know how to do this part of accepting a referral. Can someone please give me a heads up?" The next line down, someone's said, "you've made a mistake, you've mucked it up, and you know you can't do it like that". I said, "please see the previous message, which asked for some support in doing it correctly". And it got ignored, it was like, "no, we're not going to tell you how to do it". But that's evidence for me now. It's an example of where I've asked for some support with doing something, and I don't get an answer.

Chris acknowledged that documentation was time-consuming, and people, already worn down by bullying, often didn't take the time, leaving them vulnerable if anything was contested:

When you know something is happening, and it's going a particular way, you have to be really good at your documentation. That's what's so hard for many people. It's too hard. They're worn down, exhausted, not sleeping. The last thing they want to do is document what happened that day, who said what, and who was a witness. The reality is, that's the stuff they need if they ever want to formally do anything about it. In this latest situation, we had an independent review, and all I had to do was walk in and say, "these are the things that I experienced. Here's my documentation". Legally if anything was contested, I would have had to produce all that. That's why so many people leave. This is too hard.

At times careful documentation had been a source of irritation to bullies and escalated the bullying behaviour further:

I think I got more bullying because I would insist on having things on paper, and I didn't ever react. Never gave them what they really wanted. They wanted to upset me. My emails were always, "hi, how are you? just wanting to clarify this". That irritated her, but legally I was doing everything I was supposed to do. "Okay, you're telling me this. Now I just need that in writing". I was an annoyance, but I was prepared. I remember drafting an email and saying to a colleague, "I'm going to send that". And the colleague said, "are you sure you want to send that? You know that's going to aggravate them". I'm like, "yeah, I know, but legally I have to protect myself, and this is how I do that". "But you're going to make things worse for yourself". "Yeah, I probably will in the short term, but long term, I've got all the documentation I need to be able to show someone if it's ever called upon. This is what's going on. Here's the email trail".

Documentation had its challenges for Andy and Lee. Often their attempts to get things in writing were thwarted when the bully did not reply to emails:

Andy: I tried to be very clear and look at ways to avoid her reign of terror with emails to get a concrete response for evidence of what I was asked to do. But she was clever enough not to respond in that way. She might respond but not by email, so she had plausible deniability. She would say sure, do that and then be able to say I never said that. That's part of the bullies' MO. They don't want any evidence.

Lee: There were times when I was frustrated and tired because we had to do so much to work around her. You had to go back and check things and go, "Thank you very much. As per my email from the 13th", whereas when you're just collegiate and working with people usually, I go, "Oh, have you got that thing? I think I asked you for it last week".

Trying to Adapt

When things aren't good, I pull my head in and work harder. That's how I cope (Jesse).

Champions had developed many strategies to make sense of and cope with what was happening. Unfortunately, it was sometimes challenging. The shock of sudden bullying was too much for Andy, and she found herself on the back foot in dealing with it:

It was difficult because I'd never experienced it before, so I had no skill to manage someone like that. It was completely out of the blue. The other staff were feeling it too, and many left.

Chris and Jordan worked hard at compartmentalising the bullying, so they were still able to do their work and function effectively:

Chris: I was able to compartmentalise the stuff that was going on for me and still be an effective clinician with the clients I was seeing.

Jordan: I learned to become a chameleon. I tended to keep this kind of stuff to myself. I didn't want to upset other team members or burden people with my issues. So, I could walk straight out of a horrible meeting, and greet people with a smile. I used to think it was a great strength, but now I'm not so sure.

Jesse and Lee buried themselves in work to minimise the impact of bullying:

Jesse: Things you don't have control over, it's no use rallying. Why would you? One of my real gifts, and it's my Achilles heel, is that I adapt. I come from a fairly neglectful, abusive childhood. When things aren't good, I pull my head in and work harder. That's how I cope. It's actually quite debilitating because you adapt, adapt, adapt. Then you reach a point where you go, hang on, I'm only half the person I was. I've realised how bad it was now that I'm out of the situation. When I was in there, I was pushing through. I feel more traumatised about it than then because there was so much emotional stuff going on for me. I just put it in the basket, "oh yeah, I'm fine".

Lee: I don't know the name of this, but it happens to me a lot. If you're the senior one who has to hold the ship together, you come in early, follow up, and don't go for lunch. By working hard and doing these things, thinking in some small way, we can control the world a little bit.

Chris attempted to cope by learning everything she could about bullying. By understanding the motives and tactics of the bully, she was able to take the personal element out and see the situation a bit more dispassionately:

I contacted the union. I got all their information about bullying and tried to understand the behaviours and how I could cope. I did lots of reading to understand more about bullying, what it is, what it isn't, and how it can impact you. I thought the more I understood it, the more it would help. When you feel validated, "oh, yeah, this is not in my mind. This is really going on", that helps you feel better. The more I tried to understand bullying, and people's responses to bullying, the more I went; this is happening, and I did not bring this on myself. By the third time around, I knew what we were dealing with. This is not me. I'm not doing anything to deserve this. This is that person's stuff, and I'm not going to own that. So, it didn't impact me on the same level as the previous one. I wonder if it's because I had that ability to do that, that I have coped better than some people I know in similar situations. I know others who've had much more why me? What did I do to deserve that? I have that ability to go. Let's be realistic about the situation. It wasn't personal. She would have done the same thing to anyone.

Helping myself to cope when times were tough, I tried to focus on the big picture. I went to conferences often as part of my job. That made such a difference. I would often get people coming to me to thank me for my work, telling me the difference it had made to how they practised. Everyone loves an ego boost. This was so much more. It was a lifeline. It reinforced that what I was doing was worthwhile for those who matter. The crap I endured at work was devastating and unacceptable, and it didn't define me. My work defined me.

Jesse and Jordan refused to resort to their bullies' nasty and undermining tactics. Instead, they remained professional in their interactions despite how they felt deep down:

Jesse: I see him every so often, and I can't stand him. But I've never actually backstabbed him. I've never said, "Oh, this man's a complete whatever". It's just not my style.

Jordan: I am always pleasant to bullies. I say hello and pass pleasantries as I do with anyone. I do this to show that I am better than them and because I refuse to be intimidated. Although, I must admit I'm a bit naughty. I have found that my pleasant disposition drives the bullies spare. They know I am having a go, but what can they do? Complain that I am being nice to them? I do find it quite powerful.

Self-care

> I was trying to exercise and go on walks. I was trying to keep socialising. I was trying to keep doing the things I knew I liked. But I was finding it hard (Rory).

The devastating and pervasive effects of bullying can be totally absorbing, and targets may not have the motivation or the energy to take good care of themselves. The champions were no exceptions. Some took clear steps to take care as best they could. Chris was very aware that self-care was essential in helping her get through her bullying experiences:

> Checking in with my supportive people, taking the dog for a walk, and making sure I don't allow my brain or mind to think only about bullying. It will become all-consuming if you let it. I did my usual things, like going out on the weekends and going away with friends. I did mindfulness and singing. I like to sing, go to karaoke, singing at home.

Although Chris knew how important this was, it wasn't easily achieved, especially without the help of others:

> Probably truthfully, some of that would have been my mum saying, "come on, we're going away this weekend". Otherwise, I mightn't have gone. It's not like I'd consciously ring up all my mates, and we can go away together. It's much, much harder. You're in that hyper-vigilant state all the time, so when you're engaging in self-care, not really enjoying any of it, just surviving, treading water.

Taylor's experience was similar. She did prioritise self-care as much as possible and found some, although limited, benefits:

> I saw my psychologist regularly and shared with my partner, who was very supportive. I meditated, and without disclosing to people who could have influenced or knew the person involved, I sought affirmation from past colleagues and friends about my capabilities and value and worth.

I asked Taylor if the strategies were helpful:

> Yes, but only to a small degree. When you've been very traumatised in the past, if you're not feeling heard, not being supported, and not being validated by the people involved, it's really hard for those self-help strategies to have any useful degree of impact. What has sustained me has been keeping my eye on the advocacy and human rights prize and hearing and reading about the tribulations of great advocates and activists. This helps me see that bullying and intimidation aren't just about what has happened to me. Then it doesn't feel so personal, and what other people think about me or what I think about myself doesn't cause such destructive damage.

Pat also tried counselling and was unsure of how helpful it had been given that she was dealing with other issues at the same time. However, validation of her skills and competence by her peers was very valuable:

> I had some relationship stuff going on, so the counselling covered both areas. I've got a friend I went to school with. She is an outstanding social worker. She lectures and speaks at conferences, very experienced, and I'm in awe of her. She said, "Pat, you've still got those skills. You're still a good social worker". It's helpful because it stops me for a minute, and I reflect on what I'm doing.

Rory also spoke about how difficult it was to maintain self-care and keep doing what she enjoyed. On advice, she tried mindfulness and found that particularly challenging:

> I was trying to exercise and go on walks. I was trying to keep socialising. I was trying to keep doing the things I knew I liked. But I was finding it hard. I was playing lots of sport and seeing a psychologist. She was trying to get me to do an hour of mindfulness a day, but it was a huge struggle. I knew I had to sit still and just wanted to move. I put on the tape that would talk you through it, and I would go directly into overthinking. My brain would immediately go to whatever thoughts I had, and I struggled to listen. Every 30 seconds, I'd say, "Rory, you haven't listened to the last 30 seconds. Try to listen". I found it really hard and don't think mindfulness is something I will ever be great at.

Rory did receive some valuable suggestions from her counsellor that helped her cut down her alcohol consumption:

> She had previously been an Occupational Therapist and was very into utilising sensory experiences. Alcohol wasn't a big issue, but I used it to relax. So, she suggested that instead of having a gin and tonic, drink cold tonic water when you come home and see if it had the same effect. And I thought, sure, I'll try, but that won't work. But then I tried it, and it was exactly the same cold, fizzy hit. It was very surprising.

I also struggled with self-care. I knew what I should do too well, and making it happen was a huge challenge. Counselling was my most effective strategy, although sadly, I left it longer than I should have. To anyone going through bullying, my first, second, and third recommendation would be counselling. As many of us do, I thought I could and should be able to cope with this myself. Eventually, I realised I had to do something. I was in a mess. I felt completely unsupported in the workplace, and worse, I constantly felt under attack. My counsellor was absolutely fantastic. She helped me understand how I responded to bullying and how that reflected my personality type and my values. She helped me sort out what I could and couldn't control. That gave me some clarity. I realised it was never going to be even remotely the kind of working environment I needed to be able to do my job. I came to terms with the fact that the best thing for me would be to leave. I can't tell you how important that support was. She would listen to me without judgement or trying to solve everything. I honestly wish I had started counselling years before. I would've handled things differently and had more control over its impact on my life at work and home. I don't blame myself for the bullying, and the idea of counselling to sort you out, so it doesn't happen again, I don't support. Not at all.

Alex had recently commenced dialectical behaviour therapy (DBT) to assist her with the ongoing impact of her bullying experiences:

> For the longest time, I saw myself as the monster they say I am. I didn't know what emotional toll it was taking, and I'd put everything in the basket of anger and rage. Until I could identify it, I couldn't even start working on it. So, I think it is helpful, but it's going to take a while.

As well as meditation and counselling, Jesse undertook a lot of self-reflection:

> I did a lot of meditation and mindfulness. I've worked a lot on myself, and I am very good at saying this is not my problem, but I'm also good at going. Hmm, maybe this is a little bit my problem. I've been to psychologists and talked about the interactions. And why was that? And how was that? So I've tried to take something positive away from it.

Besides the counselling she was advised to have, Sam didn't take any formal measures to address her self-care. Instead, she and Andy both tried to downplay the experience as much as possible:

Sam: There is the worry that you put too much of it out there in therapy. Can you make it more real? In some ways, you're accepting that you're letting it happen. Is it really happening? or am I doing something wrong?

Andy: No counselling. I would talk to my partner or sister, reasonable people. Bounce things off. Certainly not any mindfulness. I'd try and defuse on the way home as much as I could, so I wasn't turning it over constantly at home. Trying to look at strategies and what to do to position myself. I would take some notes if I thought I should remember something, but otherwise, nothing in particular.

Chris and Jordan both used sick leave to help minimise the impact of the bullying and look after their mental health:

Chris: I would make sure I was doing my bit to look after my mental health and support those who were also struggling. And I took sick leave when I was not up to going because I didn't feel safe.

Jordan: I took sick leave. I had no trouble getting the leave. My doctor could see how stressed I was. I worked as hard, maybe harder on leave because I had a more conducive environment. People can still impact you with emails, but not as much as face-to-face. I'd have been totally justified in not working, but I had projects I wanted to finish and students I was working with. I didn't want to let people down. Besides, I really enjoyed the work. It was the environment I couldn't stand.

Shannon believed she had become resilient through learning from her first bullying experience and from facing severe health issues which altered her perspective completely:

> My whole perspective on life has changed dramatically from having cancer. I had a heart attack and broke my back, all in three years. I think that's how I've got through this, being resilient. I don't deal with bullshit, really. I'll call it and try not to let it affect me personally. I'm lucky I've got huge support and an awesome partner who lets me whinge my head off. I have a colleague in the same boat that's been my saviour. I could see how someone who wasn't in a good space, mentally, and did not have some resilience and strength about them, it could be their undoing.

6.3   Seeking Resolution

The champions wanted the behaviours to stop. They craved a positive environment where they could work harmoniously with their colleagues. They did not want to feel fearful about coming to work or anticipate how they might be bullied. To achieve this, they all sought resolution.

Taking the Informal Approach

> I know many people have bought this to you … If I put this in writing, the only person that will burn is me (Sam).

Some champions attempted to resolve their issues by going straight to the person concerned, or someone they believed could support a resolution process. When colleagues were blatantly bullied by the head of the school and her deputy, I talked to the dean of faculty. We had a solid, respectful relationship, and I could talk to him as someone who was a witness and not directly involved. I'd never seen so many dispirited people in a workplace in all my life. Most of them wouldn't have pissed down my throat if my lungs were on fire, but I have a strong sense of justice and couldn't stand by and see that behaviour continue. He told me quite frankly that he saw this as a personality clash. I said, "don't believe me, that's fine. Get somebody else to ask people". He didn't take my advice. Nothing happened until the union became involved, and there was enough evidence to support an independent inquiry. Ultimately, the bullies left, but it could and should have happened sooner. When you're in a position of authority like that it's just not okay to minimise bullying and pretend it isn't happening. If someone alerts you to a problem, you must investigate. Even if you believe it's unlikely to be true, you must. It's not ok to do nothing.

When Chris was bullied during her graduate year, she approached the nurse unit manager. Although she felt supported, she decided not to take the matter further for fear it could make things worse:

> I went to the nurse unit manager and told her I was having these experiences, and I'm pretty sure I was given a choice if I wanted to take it further. I didn't at that time. I thought it would make things worse. That's a standard response, isn't it (laughs)? How will it be for me? Back in those days, there was almost a rite of passage. We've all been there and had nurses treat us that way. You'll get used to it. You'll toughen up. It was accepted that this is what happens.

Terry went to the head of school from the university with his concerns. While she offered a potential alternative to the bullying environment, it wasn't the solution he was seeking:

> My dean was very supportive. She could pull me out of the hospital and into the school, which was a step too far because I would have come across as having failed a community leader who was the person I least wanted to disappoint.

Jordan was frustrated and concerned about the relentless bullying from the Chair and Director of the organisation. She requested mediation believing they could sort the issues as responsible adults and was stunned by what was to follow:

> I'd really had enough. There was no doubt these two had a real vendetta against me. They were trying to force me to leave the committee. I wasn't willing to do that and was determined to make this work. So, I asked for mediation. Instead, I got a request to complete a formal statement of grievance. I was shocked. I really didn't think even they would go this far. I refused to complete it. I had not made a grievance. I was trying to do the right thing and settle this between adults. What happened from there was a long-protracted process involving lawyers, investigators, a lot of money, a massive amount of time and colossal stress levels for those closely involved. When the rest of the Board was at their wit's end, it was finally agreed that the three of us would meet with two Board members to decide the way forward. Even though the purpose of the meeting was made really clear, the Chair kept pinning it on me. I had done the wrong thing and should resign. Basically, if you're not happy, resign! What a way for health professionals to behave. Ultimately the decision was that we would undertake mediation. Wasn't that what I asked for in the first place? Not once during the whole process did they do anything other than blame me. There was no "I could've done that a little better", "maybe we should've just gone straight to mediation", or "I can see how it might have affected you". I was clear that I wanted to find a way to work together. None of that ever came from them, no expressed desire for a better working relationship. To this day, it still beggars belief that two people could try so hard to use their power to get rid of somebody because they didn't like them or found them too challenging.

Leadership 101: Even if you think someone is wrong, you discuss, negotiate, and look for a win-win. Two people with senior roles in education and a professional organisation? It is bloody scary.

Pat also had her attempts at informal resolution backfire:

I remember the first time it happened. I was like, holy crap, what's going on? I went to my manager, saying, "this is what's happening. I don't appreciate being yelled at and made out that I'm not doing my job. You either have a word to her, and it stops, or I go further". So, she had a word to her, and it just made it worse, and I thought, I've had enough of this crap. I'm too old to put up with this. Life's too short.

Sam met with a senior manager to voice her concerns with little change to outcomes, so she asked a direct question to gauge whether there was support for her at that level:

I put a whole lot of stuff on the line. I said, "it's making it very hard for me to do my job. I don't understand why I'm good enough to write the model of care. I'm good enough to design wards. I have managed the best ward in the state for the last ten years, but I'm not good enough for staff recruitment anymore". I said, "Can I ask you a question, and you have to answer the honest truth? Do you want me to leave? Are you trying to get rid of me? Do you value the work I do? Because if you don't, I will go. I do a good job. We have publications, nurses involved in research, and the best ward in the state. If you don't want me to be here, I won't be here. I can't work like this".

Sam's senior manager recommended that she see a counsellor to help her develop leadership strategies to improve her relationship with her senior nurse. Although Sam didn't gain any new strategies, she did take some comfort in knowing she had done all she could:

She was telling me different ways I could respond, and I'd already tried all the things she was telling me to do, and they hadn't changed anything. So, I gave her examples. I tried the love my enemy and drive them frantic, keep my friends close and my enemies closer. I tried even being dumb and saying, "what would you do in this situation?" None of them worked. One positive thing I did come away with is that I couldn't have done anything more. I had shown her professional respect. It has not been reciprocated.

After three sessions, Sam stopped seeing the counsellor because nothing had helped. She felt uncomfortable that she was considered at fault. Finally, she told her senior manager:

I did it for three sessions. But somehow or other, it felt like I was being punished. She asked me how things were going with the counsellor. I said, "You know, strangely enough, it feels like you're punishing me. It feels like there's a problem with the two of us, but I'm the one who has to go and see someone. And I've done nothing wrong".

Sam was then encouraged by her senior manager to put her complaints in writing so that action could be taken. However, she was not confident this would make any positive difference:

She said, "If you put this in writing, I can do something about it". I was really cross with her. I said, "I know many people have bought this to you. I supervise half the people that have brought this to you. If I put this in writing, the only person that will burn is me. You will address it because you have to. Nothing will come of it".

After her performance review process, Jordan went to see the dean of faculty, her official boss, for advice and support and received the opposite of what she sought:

I was very concerned that due process for performance reviews had not been followed, and she was officially my employer. I wanted to tell her I was extremely stressed and needed advice and support. The senior nurse I depended on for funding and resources was making my job extremely difficult. During the meeting, she defended the senior nurse. Fair enough. It's her job to encourage people to see both sides of the story. She asked me to send her the relevant documentation. She offered me no advice or support. I sent her everything, radio silence! I set up a meeting with her, which was cancelled a few days before. I told her it was urgent. She blew me off, told me she had far too much going on and would get back to me when she had more time. It later became apparent why she didn't want to meet. Without my knowledge or consent, she spoke with the senior nurse and the research director. Four weeks after almost pleading for a meeting with her, I received a letter signed by the three of them via email. The letter claimed to address the concerns I had raised. Crap, it was a thinly disguised reprimand. Absolutely nothing about what the two organisations could do to support the role. I responded formally and organised another meeting. She tore shreds off me. Anything I said in my own defence was either ignored or ridiculed. When I mentioned the two years of absent or incompetent admin support, she sat back in her seat, laughed, and said, "I know all about that". I reminded her how stressful this was for me and my outrage that no one had offered or referred me to any support services. "This is a faculty of health, for goodness' sake. Shouldn't that start with looking after your staff?" She mentioned the Employer Assistance Program with no hint of concern. I realised the meeting was pointless and left.

Seeking Help Through Formal Channels

Some champions sought support and resolution through more formal channels. These actions were not taken lightly, and sadly in most cases, bad situations became worse. Lee described her reluctance to make a formal complaint because the bully had the power to put up roadblocks and make her job even harder:

The difficult thing is if you took that up to the management, you had to decide which hill to die on. The next ten things I want through this woman would be incredibly difficult. When two of our directors complained about how she impacted our team, we lost both. The message was "you can't change this". The leadership team weren't able to completely contain her.

Human Resources
I still remember a phone call from the HR manager, where he said, "I don't believe she said that to you" (Chris).

HR is generally listed as the go-to place for concerns about workplace bullying. When I completed the bullying questionnaire, the advice was to contact my HR department immediately. I laughed. I had been burned by HR. Through writing this book, reading, and engaging in social media, I discovered that very few targets of bullying received any helpful support from HR. In most cases, they got more bullying.

My own experiences with HR were mixed. At one job, I had a couple of issues. They were very helpful and supportive. Thinking about it now, though, it was when I was in favour with the organisation. When I wasn't in favour, it was a completely different matter. On one occasion, I had an issue with management. I sent all the data and an outline of my concerns to the deputy HR manager and never received a response, nothing. Overall, the champions had a very poor opinion of the support (or lack of it) from HR. Many did not believe they had the opportunity to be heard, often feeling decisions were already made:

Alex: HR asked that I have mediation with the manager. It was done by a human resource person, with no independent party. It was very, very one-sided. When I tried to say things, the HR representative would stop me and tell me that that comment wasn't appropriate or that I couldn't speak about it. It wasn't mediation. It was more of a "you're going to sit here and listen to his grievances against you". I was reprimanded for calling him a bully because it offended him. I was not allowed to use that word against him. They accused me of slandering him.

Shannon: They took the bully's side. It was all males. I had a union representative as an independent third person. They weren't very helpful because they were too busy trying to big-note themselves rather than supporting me with the issue. It didn't go well. Management wanted me to take some time off to reflect and then think about having mediation with the manager. I was the senior nurse there. I was encouraged to step back from that by HR because I wasn't shining the greatest light on professionalism, and they wanted to continue to performance manage me after that.

Chris: HR was useless as tits on a bull. It was disappointing because I thought I was doing all the right things. This is the process. This is what I do. I still remember a phone call from the HR manager, where he said, "I don't believe she said that to you". That's why the behaviour continues in health. If you get a dodgy response from HR, it's hard to go up against someone high up. It is quite rife, this behaviour within the health sector.

Terry: One of the research assistants went to HR. They did not take her seriously because it was an exit interview. They would only take her seriously if she was an employee. There have been several complaints about this person. The complaints are being ignored because the person gets grant money. The university does not care how badly you treat people as long as you get funding. That's my experience.

Lee: I was thinking about leaving by then, so I took some of this straight up to HR, who said, "Oh, yes, we're working with her and working on her, we won't allow this to happen", and yet they still did. I've been gone a couple of years now, but a similar thing happened again. When they start to tell her off, she ends up going home on stress leave, and the lawyers come, and somehow 25 years later, 26, 27 years later, whatever it is now. She's still there.

Rory: I'd gone to HR, and my initial interaction was them telling me that lots of doctors have communication and personality issues they aren't aware of. I said I've got a problem with the process and hadn't had any performance management or warnings or opportunity to respond. I didn't go back to HR for a while until I decided to make a formal complaint. It wasn't taken seriously. I never got formal acknowledgement of the complaint and had to chase everything myself. Eventually, I got a pathetic, inadequate response that basically said no, no one's done anything wrong without it having been investigated. The Employee Assistance Program got mentioned in just about every HR email. It's a great program, but it doesn't equate to HR not doing its job.

Pat: HR was on the bandwagon that I would be terminated, so they weren't willing to come to the party and help me. They said, "you're probably better off resigning". For them to terminate me was going to take about 8 weeks. I said, "i'm not coming in and putting up with this every day while you go through a process. Sack me now". They probably thought that if they did, I would take legal action, and they'd be in big trouble. I said, "you have already decided what you're going to do, so let's not play games. Sack me now". "We can't do that. You've got to resign". I went, "goodo, I'll send the email tomorrow".

Taylor: I went to HR at one point, but they thought I was mad. That I shouldn't have been working there either, so the discrimination was in HR as well.

Jesse accepted a lack of support from HR to avoid the consequence that "making waves" might have on her future job prospects:

> I did go to HR and got absolutely no support. The problem is this is a small place. I know everybody, and they all know me. You don't want to make waves in academia. So, I tentatively approached, but they were so useless. I just felt really unsupported there as well.

In one exception, Andy did have a positive experience with HR. She organised a meeting with them when her manager accused her of taking too much leave:

> The next day I said, "Let's have an appointment with HR". I called her bluff, basically. We had an appointment with HR. I said, "I'm here because my boss told me I've been red-flagged by you guys. I've had leave, but that's annual leave, long service leave. I had sick leave because I had surgery on my foot. Every single day that I've had off, apart from when my father-in-law died, I have a certificate. So, if there's a problem, let's hear it". And they said, "We have no problem with you. We have not red-flagged you". The boss didn't say anything, no reply, no apology, no response. It wasn't easy for me, but I had every right and thought I had to put a line in the sand somewhere.

Unions

> The union was as useful as hens' teeth; just was a waste of time, money and effort contacting them (Pat).

When seeking help from unions, the champions had mixed experiences. I saw one very positive outcome of union involvement when management failed to act on a complaint about bullying in the school. I let the staff use my office for a teleconference with the union because everyone else was too frightened of the repercussions if they were found out. The union surveyed staff about the workplace environment. Apart from a few sycophants, it was apparent that the environment was hostile, and bullying and favouritism were rife. That produced enough evidence for an independent inquiry. The two head bullies took advantage of timing, took redundancy packages or early retirement, and were gone. Unfortunately, we needed the union involved because management wouldn't see what was right in front of them or listen to advise, but the outcome was good.

Chris found the union helpful in providing information and advice, particularly about the difficulties she may experience in pursuing a grievance, which helped her make the decision to leave:

> The union reps were helpful. They would tell me clearly, legally, what rights I had. They were clear that this was going to be really hard. We went through all my options. They said, "if you do the thing that they're telling you in writing, you can't do, and they fire you. If you legally contest that as unfair dismissal and you win, do you really want to work somewhere where the rest of them don't really want you there? You've been tarnished as the bad egg?" And so, you weigh up all things and decide it's not worth it, just walk away.

Jordan had both positive and negative experiences:

> In one case, I was told too bad, get over it when my contract wasn't renewed under very dodgy circumstances. Another time they were fantastic, really, really supportive. The union president helped me get the best advice and support I could. At the end of the day, there wasn't a great deal I could do. I really appreciated the support, though.

Andy and Pat did not receive any helpful advice from the union to assist with the resolution of their issues:

Andy: They suggested I take sick leave. I said, "Well, that's not going to achieve anything from my perspective. It's just something I'll have to come back to and deal with when I come back". I had sick leave. I could have taken a year or 2 years off. But ultimately, it wasn't worth the stress to me.

Pat: The union was as useful as hens' teeth; just was a waste of time, money and effort contacting them. Once I said, "they are talking about performance management", they said, "nothing we can do. You've just got to go along with everything they're asking". I said, "I just need someone that's got my back to come to this meeting with me". I couldn't even get people to return my calls. I wasn't happy.

Reporting Bullying Behaviours

> I still, to this day, don't know what their expectation or purpose was other than intimidating me from ever speaking about it again (Alex).

Some champions decided to make formal complaints through a variety of channels. Finally, Shannon had enough and reported the bullying to senior management when the situation seemed totally out of hand:

> My colleague came to work a couple of weeks ago and looked really unwell. She burst into tears. She said, "I'm so cross with the girls. They've withheld this information again, and I have been hauled over the coals. And they laughed while I was being told off. I'm over it. I'm bigger than this. I don't play these games". We went to management and said we couldn't manage the situation. This is bigger than us. We don't know what we don't know. We're probably a risk to the organisation, so either we should leave, or we need a really robust policy and procedure put in place by senior management. They put it back on us: "This is performance management". I said, "I don't call it performance management. I call it bullying". Our bullying policy talks to exactly this behaviour, excluding, sniggering behind your back, setting you up to fail, and giving you the referral they know you're going to make a mistake on. The manager said, "I need individual examples". And, you know what? We came up with very few between us.

Andy provided a short and sweet account of the outcomes of her and her colleagues' attempts to address the bullying behaviour after many staff resignations:

> Those who remained wrote to head office, and they said, "Too bad, so sad".

Chris made a formal complaint after one of her bullying experiences. Participating in the complaints process clarified for her the type of person the bully was. She had no confidence in the likelihood of an amicable outcome, particularly since the bully had the backing of the organisation:

> I put in a grievance. Trying to do the right thing. And we had mediation. As a mental health nurse, it's not my job to diagnose other colleagues. Still, with some of the knowledge that I have, I was dealing with a particular type of personality structure, which meant that it was never going to be a safe place for me. I'd tried to take it up to management to say this behaviour's going on. I've got a record of this. They completely dismissed me: "we don't believe that that's going on at all, and we're going to back her".

Finding herself in another bullying and toxic environment and after trying every conceivable option, Chris contacted the Board of Management:

> I wrote an anonymous letter to the Chair. I spelled out the behaviours I'd witnessed and been informed of and how they impacted staff. Something like 10 or 12 people left because of this person. We teach other people about creating a mentally healthy workplace. I wrote the letter to say that all the things we're supposed to stand for as an organisation are currently under threat because of this person. The letter helped. There was a review, and everyone was interviewed anonymously. And the outcome was that she no longer works there.

When Lee took a similar action about her bullying concerns, there was some initial reluctance to become involved. She had to be intense and persistent before action was taken:

> Initially, they did the usual Board shit, "Oh, we're governance. That's operations. We don't want to interfere". I was like, "Mate, I'm telling you, you've got a lawsuit coming. Because if I've got to put up with a minute more of it, I'll be going to a lawyer. How are you going to look when this is your bread and butter, telling people about mentally healthy workplaces, and you have four lawsuits for bullying?"

Once they were persuaded, Lee worked with the Board to ensure the bully was dismissed:

> I was working with the Board behind the scenes. They were asking me to report back what she was saying at the meetings because she would say one thing in meetings, one thing to them and the minutes were a complete riot. So I started taking notes of the meetings. They hired a lawyer. For once, it did have a swift resolution. She was marched out of the place.

When Alex was assaulted by an educator, a colleague who witnessed the assault strongly encouraged her to report it. However, rather than the incident being investigated, Alex was subjected to more bullying across all levels of the organisation:

> "You were assaulted today. You need to call the police because nobody's doing anything". I said, "That's going to create a shit storm for me". He finally said, "If you don't report it, I'm going to", So I did. The head of department seemed quite shocked and extremely upset by what had happened. I felt maybe this is going to be okay. The next day I was called to meet with the department head, and his demeanour towards me could not have been more different. He was essentially accusing me of lying, of being the aggressor. He was intimidating me not to report it to the police. He told me I would be going outside operating procedures. I left the interview like a scolded child. I felt dehumanised. That night I just cried. I called my partner and friends and said, "I want to give up. I want to leave here". They encouraged me to stay and told me to document everything, do what they told me, and follow the operating procedures. The next morning two senior educators pulled me into this other room. They have the girl that assaulted me and other people in the room. There were brass and buttons and uniforms, and it was very scary. They told me I was expected to straight-talk her. That is their policy. You're supposed to confront the other employee about the behaviour. I was frozen. I didn't know what to do. I didn't know what to say. I just wanted out of the room as quickly as I could. It was one of the most uncomfortable positions I've ever been in. It would be like if you were in an abusive relationship and the police pulled in your spouse and said, "All right, straight talk". I don't know how they expected me to correct the situation; I was powerless. I wanted out of the room so badly that I became very amiable and brushed off the whole situation saying, "it's not that big a deal". I still, to this day, don't know what their expectation or purpose was other than intimidating me from ever speaking about it again.

As Alex feared, the bullying behaviour became worse from that point and quickly turned to mobbing:

> Her allies in the class made my life a living hell every day. They attempted another straight talk. I refused to go into the room. I said, "I'm not doing it. I am emotionally and mentally exhausted. I need to finish my studies and exams and take care of myself". The department

head became enraged, and a senior educator told me I had failed to follow standard operating procedures. They were refusing to investigate any claim about the assault any further. They were closing that case. It did not exist to them anymore.

Alex turned to her supervisor for support and assistance when all efforts failed. The outcome was not what she expected:

> I went to my peer support officer, who was also my supervisor. I told him that mentally I was not coping, being in the same environment as this woman. I was trying to have my roster set up so I didn't have to see her. I thought he was a peer support officer. Surely to God, he's going to do something. It seemed like putting blood in the water with sharks. It was like, this girl is weak. We're going to attack her. He did everything he could to ensure that any request I made to alleviate the situation was denied. They scheduled me for the second leg of training. I said, "I cannot go back to that place. I'm having nightmares; I'm not sleeping". He said, "everybody has to work with people they don't like at some point. You need to grow up". I said, "This isn't me not wanting to work with someone I dislike". He said, "Well, you have to give me a better reason than what you're giving me", I said, "You need a better reason than assault? Does she have to kill me? What is going to make you listen to me? I want to be relieved of any further educational requirement". He told me he would make a notation on the official file that I had family issues and could not continue. I said, "I'm not going to sign that". He said he would give me a permanent role as a call-taker where I would not dispatch the emergency resources. That offer was rescinded, and I had to go back to training.

When a new person became her supervisor, the situation escalated further:

> I could tell from the first meeting that he had already been briefed on me. He was very hostile. He gritted his teeth and his finger in my face when talking to me. They started refusing to approve my timesheet. For well over a month, I wasn't paid. When I went to the union, they stopped approving my partner's timesheet. The union filed with the Industrial Relations Court, and on the day the hearing was to take place, they finally approved my timesheets.

The harassment even followed her at home during periods of sick leave:

> I said I wouldn't be in. I always provided a doctor's certificate. My supervisor would call me to confront me about why I wasn't coming to work. I got so tired of it. I actually swore one day and hung up on him. He came to my house to confront me, and I asked him to leave. After that, he would come to my house anytime he wanted to confront me. I emailed our professional standards and conduct unit and asked them for help. They told me I needed to approach my supervisor and try to come to an understanding with him about it.

After receiving no assistance from within the organisation, Alex went to the police:

> I finally went to the police. One thing they threw at me was that I had never reported the initial assault. They're acting like it never happened. They have no record. One of the executives who knows what happened and feels really horrible sent me a copy of the file. I can't use it because it would cost her job. I filed a police report, and the lady who took my report said, "I want you to know that I believe you. I know what that place does to their employees". I was so thankful. I thought, "oh my God, somebody's going to do something". She went on maternity leave, and it got transferred. Even though I have a witness statement that

was very, very detailed about dates, times and what happened, the police officer told me he had spoken to the head of department, who had satisfied him that nothing had ever happened to me. I said, "I've got emails and messages I can send you. I've got all this information. He said, 'That's so old. I can't accept any of that'. I asked him to pull the files and have them subpoenaed?" He said, "I'm not going to do that". He told me he was closing the case that day, and he did.

Rory described the lengthy process that followed her complaint:

I went to my mentor initially, then to the director and then HR. I contacted the chief medical officer, who didn't respond. I went to other people above the director. Other people were hearing about it but weren't communicating with me. I'd already been speaking to the complaints people within my training college, but they couldn't help. I eventually contacted the president of the college. I told him what had happened. He told me he would contact the hospital and get back to me. He did contact them. He told me he would contact them again in a week, which I believe he did. And then, he never got back to me, despite my contacting him. They've also blocked my email, so I can't email the hospital.

After her suicide attempt, learning her employment offer had been rescinded, and with no means of communicating with people from the hospital, Rory's parents wrote to the health department expressing their concerns:

They asked for an investigation. It took the department four and a half months until they collected enough information to know the hospital staff hadn't answered any of the questions, and they needed to investigate further.

Rory did eventually receive her requested documents through freedom of information. There were literally hundreds of emails between HR, supervisors, and senior medical staff. Rory talked about the most important ones that clearly demonstrate the decision to retract their offer of employment for reasons that were clearly personal and the efforts they took to protect themselves from possible industrial relations actions:

There are many emails from after I left, and they decided to retract the job offer. There are emails from the Director of ED where they're given the final decision of whether to retract the job offer, and they say yes. Then emails between HR and the chief medical officer where they recommend specific wording to say it is due to funding. There is blatant evidence that it's not due to funding. The chief medical officer didn't want to respond, saying, "do we even have to do this? We didn't give her a formal contract". HR said I needed a response because I'd been given the offer in writing. There are probably at least a handful of times where they mention they're worried about it becoming an industrial relations issue. Clearly, their intention is to silence me rather than deal with it.

The process of waiting for further information was frustrating; it was moving very slowly, and communication was not always forthcoming:

The last I heard, the health department would look into how Hospital HR managed my complaint and how I was treated. They can't give me any timeframes. They told me they would try to give me updates every fortnight, but it hasn't happened, mainly because they don't have anything to update me on. I was told they'd written a letter to the appropriate person at the hospital, and they've received information back, which is being reviewed. I'm just waiting. That was six weeks ago. It's been really hard. It just feels like I'm going through bullying and intentional obstruction. I can't really think about it any other way. I'm trying to be as patient as I can.

I asked Rory what outcomes she would like at the end of this process:

I want repercussions for the people who did this to me. I want some people to lose their jobs. I want a formal apology from the health department. I don't care for one from the hospital because I don't think they're sorry. I want my job back. I want a promise that I can go back whenever I want.

Somewhat surprised, I asked if she would go back, given the option:

Yes. I went there last week to visit my friends, and I missed it, and I wanted to be back there, and I get that, logically, that makes no sense. But yes.

Legal Advice
You've got a really good case … I can certainly represent you. But obviously, I've got to pay. And I just thought, no, by then, I didn't have the energy for it.

Shannon considered taking legal action, but after receiving advice, she realised it wasn't an affordable or emotionally advisable option to take it further:

I spoke to a lawyer friend, and she said, "You've got a really good case if you want to do it. You've got all these women saying that he's a sexual predator. I can certainly represent you". But obviously, I've got to pay. And I just thought, no, by then, I didn't have the energy for it.

Nowhere to Turn
I went to human rights, and they said, "It's got to be a bit more than what's happening" … "What? I have to have a nervous breakdown first before you pay attention?" (Pat).

At the end of all their efforts, some champions were left feeling utterly unsupported with nowhere to go for assistance:

Pat: There was nowhere. Every government organisation I rang said, "Oh, it's the government. We can't help. You've got to go to your union". So, you go to the union, and they're not interested. So I went to human rights, and they said, "It's got to be a bit more than what's happening", and I'm like, "What? I have to have a nervous breakdown first before you pay attention?"
Rory: Other colleagues spoke to me about going to my professional organisations. All of which I did, none of whom could help.

6.4   Leaving or Staying?

I lost a lot by leaving financially, socially, and professionally. Those two managers would have been the two to give me a reference … that wasn't something I would ever ask them to do (Shannon).

I often hear "just leave", "nothing is worth your mental health" from articles I read, social media, and in life more broadly. Really? I suspect the mental health implications of losing the house or being unable to feed and clothe the kids would be pretty high too. Finding a new job isn't always that easy, and there is the issue of getting a good reference from the current one. I was heartbroken at leaving jobs I loved because of what others did to me. I had moved interstate twice, so it wasn't just about leaving the job. It was uprooting a life and starting up another. Deciding whether to leave a job is highly complex. Most champions had left their job, and those still in the bullying environment wanted to leave:

Shannon: I feel totally powerless now. It's a fight that I don't feel I should have to have. I refuse to take on that extra stress. It's not what my health needs. I feel I am forced to leave because there is no intervention, and I won't put myself through it anymore.

Andy: I didn't know how to manage her because she was off her fucking tits. I didn't have the skills to cope with her, and so I ended up just leaving, which is what tends to happen. Not many people can stand up for that sort of thing. So I thought I might as well find something else I can do, and you can have it, which is quite disappointing. You work hard, get a reasonable job that pays well, and go, "No, it's too hard".

This disappointment was shared by others making the same often heartbreaking decision to leave. Unfortunately for Jordan, it became a pattern that would emerge over time and result in her leaving jobs she had previously loved:

So, I left. I loved the job, but I couldn't handle the working environment anymore. Work is such an essential part of what I do and who I am that it just isn't an option to coast along, only do what I have to and keep quiet in the background. So, I left the next job, the one after, and the one after that. Although one of them was not entirely my choice, I was going anyway. It was all because of bullying and toxic environments. The unfortunate thing is I'm sure that all my bullies were delighted to see me go, even though I was good at my job and very successful. I would never suggest I didn't make mistakes and there weren't things I could learn. That's the problem with subtle bullying. It doesn't allow you to learn and change. No one will be honest and admit they have a problem with you. Instead, they make your life more and more difficult, so you'll leave, and so I did. I was over it. And after that first job, the cycle began. I would have long periods of working in a really positive environment. I was productive and happy. Then someone would leave, and the new person would dislike me. I was lucky I didn't have difficulty getting a new job, but it frustrated me. I've seen it so often with others that they either leave or hibernate quietly in the corner; either way, their potential isn't realised.

Shannon took extended leave and later resigned. It was a very difficult decision to leave her job, and it came at a considerable cost. However, she felt the reputational damage was too great to return:

I was angry. I didn't want to have to face them. I felt like I would face the music when I got back. That I was in a firing line already. I don't think it would have mattered how well I had contributed to the team, management, or practice. I was still in the firing line because there was unfinished business. So, I had about 12 months off. I hadn't intended to finish up there, but I did. It's a bittersweet pill. I didn't have a goodbye after 18 years. I wanted to hit my 20 years and go out on a hoorah. I felt really ostracised because I wasn't there. I just felt judged by everyone. And you never know what's being said once you're out the door. I took a hit to my reputation. I lost a lot by leaving financially, socially, and professionally. Those two managers would have been the two to give me a reference at that time. And that wasn't something I would ever ask them to do.

There was some satisfaction for Shannon when she hit back at the bully and successfully had the complaint against her withdrawn:

> The day before I went on leave, I walked into the manager's office and gave him the opportunity to either withdraw his complaint or I had 25 signed Stat Decs from female staff, who all had their own incidents with him. Here was the proof in the pudding. So, he withdrew the complaint. He showed me he had deleted the email and gave me the USB with all the paperwork. I took the USB, gave him the Stat Decs and watched him shred them in front of me.

I asked Shannon why she left after the complaint was withdrawn:

> I didn't have support. I was seen as an instigator and considered a liar. It was very hurtful. When it was time to come back, I was triggered because I was never followed up when I was away. I didn't know what I was going to walk into.

Sam loved her job and had been working there for a long time. So the thought of leaving was devastating, both emotionally and financially:

> What do I do? I need money. Do I work privately for someone forever? It's boring. So, it's looking for something else to do when you've been on the job for a long time. It is a hard line between loving my job because I may have to think about not doing the thing I love.

Deciding to resign was complicated for Pat. She was in considerable debt after a long illness. She was also worried that her age would pose a barrier to getting a new job:

> At the time, I was still paying off my car, I had rent, and credit card bills to pay. The recruitment guy would say they're really interested in interviewing you. I said, "yeah, because I look really good on paper, I'm a 55-year-old woman". I'm up against new grads. One would think I'd be looking good to an employer because I've had babies, so I'm not going to take time off to have babies, but apparently not. They still want the young ones.

Ultimately, she did leave, but not voluntarily. Performance management was the ultimate tool, leaving Pat feeling powerless:

> My boss rang me. "Are you coming in?" I said, "No". "You should have rung, and you haven't followed policy". I said, "I spoke to the senior social worker yesterday and told her I wouldn't be coming in". I was in the car on hands-free, and I raised my voice so she could hear. When I went back to work, I was called into a meeting with another manager, and he said, "She feels intimidated by you because you yelled at her on the phone". I thought, seriously? She's bullying me, and I have told you that she's bullying me. It kept going. I approached the executive level of the organisation and said, "look, I'm being bullied". And as soon as I said I was being bullied and had contacted the union, it switched. Now I was

being performance managed. I got some pro bono legal advice through the Cancer Council. They said, "because it's performance management, there's really nothing you can do". HR said "If you're performance managed. We terminate you if you go for any other job and they ring; we've got to let them know that. If you resign and go for another job and they ring, we're not allowed to say anything about you being performance managed". My hands were tied. I had to resign, and that's what I did.

Despite finding the bullying unbearable, Andy refused to leave. Having left a very good job because of bullying, she wasn't prepared to do it again:

Rightly or wrongly, I had that sense of, well, fuck you. As miserable as this is, I will not lose my job again or have to do something else I don't want to do because of you. What this job provides is that we are still within the public hospital system with all my entitlements, which are quite significant. It gives me a virtual Monday-to-Friday job and extra cash for being on call. It gives me six weeks' holiday a year. It's a very rare thing, and I like what I do. I did not like her, and I felt, from the previous experience, why should I lose my job because of you? Why should I have to? So, I didn't.

Terry was torn, wanting to leave the toxic environment and being hampered because he had travelled from his home country to take up the job. Unfortunately, it wasn't so easy to turn around and go back:

Being in a new country and a new role gets to me, and I'm worried at many different levels. Had this been at home, I would have just left the position a long, long time ago. But it's so expensive to come here, to go back again. I'm here. I'm on one of the adventures of my life, but it has become part of my worry, and I can see that this is taking up so much energy.

I have a right to voice my opinion. Others don't have to agree. They have an obligation to listen. If people listened to hear rather than dismiss or belittle, we could all make a greater contribution (Jordan).

Why is this happening to me? The champions found themselves asking this question time and time again. When the issue of why me came up in our conversations, I was clear that this wasn't about responsibility or blame. I wasn't asking what the champions had done to cause bullies to behave and act the way they did. Bullying is the responsibility of the bully. If you have been bullied, please, please remember this always. I get tired of reading social media messages suggesting targets should "refuse" to be bullied. "Stop complaining about people who are draining you when you keep handing them the straw" is particularly offensive and completely missing the point. It would hardly be bullying if targets could say, "Please don't do that", and the bully would respond, "I'm sorry I didn't realise I had upset you". Speaking that way to a bully may result in worse behaviours, with the target being seen as confrontational or vulnerable.

Suggesting the target is somehow to blame or is in control of the situation does not reflect the power inequities and broader cultural issues that allow bullying to continue. It doesn't reflect the subtle bullying the champions described in *Bully Tactics*.

To understand "why me", we must look beyond the schoolyard bully who picks on the weak. Research suggests the opposite is more likely. People who are competent, hardworking, well respected, honest, and assertive are more likely to be targeted by bullies who feel threatened by their success and popularity. Sadly, bullies often target members of their team, people whose hard work and achievements would benefit the organisation and reflect positively on the bully. My conversations with the champions brought many of these reasons we read about to life. Many resonated with my experiences.

© The Author(s), under exclusive license to Springer Nature
Switzerland AG 2024
B. Happell, *Sickness in Health: Bullying in Nursing and other Health Professions*, https://doi.org/10.1007/978-3-031-49336-2_7

7.1   Gentle Nature

I think bullies feel stronger than people who show any fragility or vulnerability. They feel safer attacking people who are gentler than they are (Taylor).

Taylor described herself as gentle-natured and saw bullies as stronger people, preying on the weak or kind, much like the schoolyard bully:

There are types of us that are bullied more easily. People who are gentler are bullied. I think bullies feel stronger than people who show any fragility or vulnerability. They feel safer attacking people who are gentler than they are. That's where it happens. If you carry yourself confidently, people are less likely to bully and intimidate you.

7.2   Assertive and Outspoken

This person's behaviour changed towards me when I started to really challenge the behaviour and say, this is not okay (Chris).

Taylor demonstrated her gentle nature throughout our conversations. However, she also revealed she was very capable of standing up to bullying behaviour, particularly when protecting the rights of patients:

A patient had accused a doctor of being a paedophile. I took that to the police. Doctors and nurses abused me, pinned me in the room, flicked me on the end of the nose, and called for my sacking. He yelled and yelled and yelled at me. I'm not good at advocating for myself. When they stopped yelling, they said, "Now, what have you got to say for yourself?" I just said, "Me thinks thou dost protest too much". There's a point where they push and push you, and it's uncomfortable and awful. Then they become ridiculous. And they had stepped over that line. And that made me feel stronger in going to defend her. The doctor ended up in jail, and the patient turned their life around, and I got stronger with it.

Rory and Jesse also found themselves targets of bullying when they stood up for the rights of others:

Rory: I had said something to someone who was bullying another staff member, and they didn't like that. I have a strong sense of what I think is right and wrong, which gets me into trouble.

Jesse: It's a lot about "I need to put you down because I need to build myself up". I will intervene and say, "Hang on, you can't treat someone like that. You can't do that". That doesn't go down well.

Being assertive, as I am, can be either an asset or a liability, depending on whether you are in favour of those who hold power or not. It is astounding that expressing a different opinion or questioning an action or decision could unleash a bully. It frustrates and bewilders me for health professionals, whose focus should also be improving health services and outcomes. It is unconscionable for academics who are supposed to respect and uphold freedom of speech. Chris, Pat, and Jesse described themselves as assertive and outspoken, characteristics not welcomed by the bullies:

Chris: One of the reasons she didn't like me is because I was a stickler for the rules. She'd ask me to check something, and I'd say, but I haven't seen you draw it up, so I can't check that medication. And she'd roll her eyes, get annoyed. There was a lot of "Who are you? You're this young thing, you've just come out of uni, and you should just do what you're told". I wasn't prepared to do that. I was always okay about saying no when I thought I'd be doing something wrong by saying yes.

Chris: This person's behaviour changed towards me when I started to challenge the behaviour and say, this is not okay. I'd point to inconsistencies in their communication and would try and have everything documented. Once this person had worked out that I'd really got their number, the person embarked on a bit of a mission to get rid of me. The second I stood up to all her stuff, I knew my days were numbered. I was no longer of any use to her. In fact, I was now a threat because I was actively showing others her behaviours. I've gone to management, and I've gone to her boss, and then higher up. I became a threat because I was trying to bring to other people's attention to the behaviour that was not okay.

Jesse: He was a man that needed everybody to agree with him, and I'm not good at that. If someone's wrong, I'll say, "Well, yeah, I think that's probably wrong". He was the font of all wisdom. No one should say no to him. Most of the staff were really on board. He thought he knew everything and that he should be obeyed mindlessly.

Pat: While I was away, they employed a new grad to cover my position. The manager had organised this new grad to mentor me. I said, "No, I'm not being mentored by a new grad. Find somebody with a couple of years of experience. Not the new grad sucking up your backside because I won't do that". I don't crawl or grovel for anyone.

Because Taylor and Jordan stood up for their convictions, others saw them as enjoying confrontation for the sake of it. This seemed to further irritate bullies who did not welcome open discussion and differing opinions:

Taylor: Because I'm an activist, people think I like confrontation. I hate it, really hate it. This is about human rights. That's why I'm fighting this.

Jordan: I'm not confrontational for the sake of it. I have strong values and principles. I put myself forward for committees and working groups because I believe I have something to contribute. I'm not interested in padding my CV. I feel a responsibility to contribute actively to committees or groups I am a member of. At times that means I have different opinions from others in the group. I will say what I think. Often that is fine, understood and probably respected. At other times it's as though people think I've only turned up to cause trouble. That couldn't be more wrong. I had serious concerns about the actions of a staff member of the organisation. As a management committee member, I voiced those concerns. I was ignored by the Chair. Serious issues with the staff member and the broader organisation were eventually revealed and worse than expected. A long, tortuous process followed before we could deal with the problems and get the organisation back on track. One committee member came to me after a particularly lengthy and draining meeting and said he owed me an apology. He said: "When you first came onto this committee, I thought you were a pain in the arse, arguing for the sake of it and giving the director a hard time because you didn't like her, and now I understand that everything you said was right". It was a sincere and most welcome apology. Not surprisingly, I didn't receive anything like that from the Chair. It's never personal. It's not for kicks. I don't understand why people are offended by a well-reasoned argument or a different point of view. I have a right to voice my opinion. Others don't have to agree. They have an obligation to listen. If people listened to hear rather than dismiss or belittle, we could all make a greater contribution.

7.3   Seen as Threatening

Imagine being so small that you've got to dump on someone else to make yourself big (Jesse).

Feeling threatened is, unfortunately, very common in managers and entirely at odds with good leadership. One manager's attitude changed when I completed my master's degree. It was when very few nurses had master's degrees in universities. She was not one of them. On one occasion, when dressing me down, she said, "You may have academic qualifications, but you lack life experience". The stupid thing is I did not care less that she didn't have a master's degree. She had a lot of experience in management and education in the hospital system, and she deserved that job. I wasn't interested in her job anyway.

On another occasion, after starting a new job, I went to a meeting at a drug and alcohol service. I had previously worked in that field and knew most of the staff. It was a very small world. I was asked if I wanted to join a conference organising committee. I later learned that my former boss had been asked to nominate a staff member with a background in drug and alcohol while I was working there. When I heard the name of the person nominated, I was gobsmacked. She had no experience in drug and alcohol or mental health either. At the time, I was doing drug and alcohol research with a partner health service, so there is no way my manager did not know about my background. What kind of a person does that? You must feel awfully threatened when you prefer to send someone who is part of your inner circle even though someone else is much more suitable.

Jesse's first bullying experience came after applying for the same job as her boss. Even though he was successful, he clearly felt very threatened by her. The tension between them was ongoing and intensified:

I was surprised that he could not get above the fact that I'd also applied for the job and didn't get it because I was definitely not trying to undermine him. He decided to come on the attack, thinking I would try to undermine him, but that has never really been who I am.

He was not of interest to me. So that was, I guess, unflattering. It was never about him for me, but obviously, it was a little bit about me for him.

For Jesse, the ongoing bullying was about her boss's ego, which shielded his underlying weakness and vulnerability. By bullying her, he felt able to enhance his own self-esteem:

Oh my God. It's about ego. It was just so personal. The fact he said I was threatening was hilarious because I wasn't threatening at all. I still think he's the biggest bastard on earth. I was just appalled. I don't know how people like that live in the world. How can he get away with people really liking and respecting him, and he's just so awful? He's an awful, awful person. Imagine being so small that you've got to dump on someone else to make yourself big. I was so pleased to get away from him, and I loved that I got away from him, and I probably would've rather been unemployed than have gone back.

Jesse saw this experience as one example of an ongoing pattern of bullying she faced because she was productive and successful, which threatened her far less successful bosses:

She was threatened by me because I had many more publications than her, and she did have a bit of a complex. I felt bullied by her. I stood in for her as director while she went overseas. Unfortunately, I did too good a job. She actually said to me, "You made it look like I do nothing". Her main job was going out to coffee with people. And I'm not a big coffee drinker. I prefer to work. So, I did my job, and her job still managed to run the place and had no problems. So, she had to find things to have a go at me about. She had to find issues later.

Similarly, Jordan had a boss who seemed to see her as a potential competitor. Jordan felt her boss was worried that because of her qualifications and achievements, she may have her eye on the boss's job:

A new head of school was appointed; academically, I was much more qualified than her. I was developing a publication track record and had PhD students. She had none. I couldn't care less. I didn't want her job. I just wanted to have a decent working relationship with her. Unfortunately, that didn't happen; she did everything possible to hamper my success. The only reason I can think of is she felt threatened.

Chris saw her bully boss as expecting unconditional loyalty for her leadership. When she could no longer count on this loyalty, their relationship suddenly changed from collegial to adversarial:

Many people were on the receiving end of lots of behaviour, but three or four of us copped the most. And it's hard to know, was that because, for some reason, I was dobbed in by someone to say I didn't like the leadership? She had this mindset. You're either for me or against me. So, had she heard this whisper from someone I was against her? "I'm going to make her life difficult" because you're either on the bus or under the bus.

Jordan believed she was a target for bullying in a broader professional role. The committee Chair was clearly not open to questions or differing opinions and described alternative points of view as challenging her leadership:

The Chair said to me on more than one occasion that she would not have her leadership challenged. I could barely ask a question or offer an opinion without being accused of challenging her leadership. How is asking a question that I have a right and a responsibility to ask challenging leadership? Real leaders welcome differing opinions. That is what makes them leaders. She was more like a dictator. I find that attitude utterly bewildering and inappropriate in any situation. Coming from a health professional takes it into a whole new league, and I find it scary. Don't people, particularly health professionals, realise that if you need to stamp your authority, you are not a leader? There is something wrong, and you need to deal with it. I learned that lesson early. I consciously told myself that if I needed to silence or admonish someone for expressing an opinion, I might not like, it's time to get help or get out.

Sam was saddened that the bully could not see the detrimental impact of her behaviour on the service:

The team I am blessed to be part of is performing, and we are recognised nationally and internationally. Why wouldn't you embrace that and own it for your own ego rather than try and destroy it? That's what I don't understand. She's threatened by me. But I don't know why. If I were in her position, I would look at the areas that are doing really well and own them as my own.

Pat and Lee believed the bully they worked with felt threatened by several staff or even the team they inherited when they started the job. The need to feel secure and in control was so strong they worked towards dismantling the existing cohesive staff profile and creating an entirely new team:

Pat: I think, and now more so because other people have resigned, that she wants to create her own team because we'd had that team for probably close to 8, 10 years, and everybody had each other's back. I think she wanted to make her own team with people she had chosen and could manipulate. I think she looked at me and thought, "Oh well, she's coming back from illness. She's not going to stay long. She'll go". "Well, no, I'm not going, I'm staying", maybe that was the reason. Perhaps she thinks she's clearing out the old workforce, or she's had directions from the CEO to get rid of the workers who have been there longer. I don't know, but I think she's trying to get her own army.

Lee: Suddenly, we lost senior, experienced people who were brilliant at their work, and we had this bunch of 26, 28, 32-year-olds who were nice enough but had no experience in education or training, no understanding of the system. I think that's what she wanted, people who were not skilled, underlings. We'd just gotten rid of 30 staff who had at least 15 years of clinical experience in mental health. Some new staff produced work, and I told management, "This kid was supposed to send this thing out. It's a big project, 800 grand for training. She's written this thing and it was, like, a random bunch of shit she'd put together". When I brought this up to leadership and said, "I'm really concerned. Somebody needs to be supervising. We need to go back through all her work". I got the kicking, not her.

7.4 Honesty

I'm very honest. Bullies struggle with the truth. So, if I'm just going to tell you the truth, they're, like, whoa, hang on, I don't think we deal in the truth here, do we (Jesse)?

Champions who valued honesty were seen as challenging to bullies who did not appreciate a direct and open approach. I can certainly relate to that. I say what I think—that's who I am. I generally tell people I'm direct, open, and honest and value that in others. Lots of people say they appreciate that, and they really don't. I don't understand it. I would much rather have someone say, "I don't agree", or "I don't like that", or "I think it is wrong", than have them smile and nod and be resentful or bag me to other people. I'm not asking people to agree or take any action. I want my right to say what I think to be respected and not admonished. Surely in an academic environment, particularly health, that should be respected.

Taylor and Jesse talked about bullies being unable to deal with honest people, making them a target on many occasions:

Taylor: People are really afraid of honesty. They're really afraid of people who do speak honestly. They want everybody to just toe the line, be mundane, be vanilla. Anything that supports their position in life, society, and the workplace, that's what they want. They can't cope with anybody being honest about anything different to their perspective, their point of view.

Jesse: I interact differently to other people, and can look a bit challenging. One of my problems is I'm very honest. Bullies struggle with the truth. So, if I'm going to tell you the truth, they're, like, "Whoa, hang on, I don't think we deal in the truth here, do we?"

When Andy spoke of her first bullying experience, she was still confused many years later about why the bully chose to target her. Because Andy had acted in the bully's role before her appointment, she wanted to be clear from the outset that she had not been interested in the position. She wanted to demonstrate her commitment and let the boss know she bore no resentment. Her honesty cost her dearly:

I don't know whether she thought I had a bit of resilience and could push back or I was a weak link? I don't know. She didn't know me when it started. It was only a couple of weeks in when I thought okay, I will just let you know, "I wasn't after your job. I am here to support you". And then it was on, really. I don't know. I honestly don't know.

7.5 Well Respected

I'm not everybody's favourite, but I'm pretty much 90% respected by the people I'm responsible for (Sam).

Chris, Sam, and Jordan described themselves as well respected and generally well liked by their peers. They believed the bullies felt the need to "bring them back to size", despite the valuable contributions they made:

Chris: In the positions that I've been in, I did get along with others, I was well
          liked, and I believe I was really good at my job.
Sam: I'm not everybody's favourite, but I'm pretty much 90% respected by the
          people I'm responsible for. I'm sure they talk behind my back and say
          I'm a bitch when they didn't get that extra staff member. But I think, for
          the most part, I'm very well respected.
Jordan: Responses to me at a personal level are mixed. Some people see me as a
          hard-arse and unreasonable bitch. Most have never worked with me or no
          longer benefit from my collegiality. I do have a solid professional reputa-
          tion. I am considered a significant leader in my field, with tall poppy
          syndrome alive and well in healthcare that pisses some people off. It is
          easier to hate me than appreciate what I have contributed.

7.6   Hard Workers

> I doubled the training and the income in one year … while being bullied. "What do you
> think I could fucking do if you actually supported me (Lee)?"

I can certainly relate to this. I've always been a hard worker. You would think
intuitively that that would be a protective factor against bullying. It certainly wasn't
in my case, and I have seen so often people ingratiating themselves to managers
getting a lighter load or unwarranted promotions. In one job, many of my colleagues
would whinge and moan about their workloads while playing computer solitaire in
their office. They got the easy ride. I had more and more work poured onto me to
compensate. Sometimes I'd think my life would be much easier if I was more like
them, just did what had to be done and nothing more. That's just not me. If I do a
job, I want to be proud of it. I have always found it distasteful that the whingers
coast through, and the hard workers get to pick up the slack.

My experience was not unique. Jesse and Lee described being bullied because of
their hard work. It was also a source of incredible frustration that the bullying hampered their ability to achieve even more.

Jesse: I'm an easy target because I am so conscientious. I work hard and push
          through stuff. Oh, well, I'm just going to do this anyway.
Lee: I doubled the training and the income in one year with both hands tied
          behind my back while being bullied. You want to say to them, "What do
          you think I could fucking do if you actually supported me?" Oh, my
          serious God.

Chris and Andy felt particularly blindsided by bullying because they had always
been valued as staff, and no performance issues had been raised previously:

Chris: I'd always been a highly valued employee. All my performance appraisals
          were amazing. So, to have, what I considered, the higher-up of the organ-
          isation thinking you're a bad egg. We want you gone, oh my God, that's
          going to take me a moment to get my head around.

Andy: I felt that, as someone senior in the organisation, I had done my job very
         well, and I had had no clue, no feedback from any other managers before
         her that I wasn't doing the job that I should be doing.

7.7   Punishment

> I said things that were very uncomfortable for them to hear, and they never wanted anyone
> to hear. They're going to punish me for that … make an example of me (Alex).

Andy, Alex, Chris, and Terry interpreted bullying behaviour as punishment for
actions or inactions the bully disapproved of. When Andy's boss discovered she had
spoken to the union, their relationship changed dramatically. Andy's attempts to
explain that she had purely been seeking information were in vain:

Andy: She was upfront that she was pretty fucking pissed off with me. Even
         though I explained to her, that's not what was meant to have happened. I
         wanted to know where I stood as a union member. I've gone home, and
         there's no roster for my next week time and time again. I don't want my
         boss to be pissed off at me because I've already experienced that before. I
         wanted to find some strategies and skills because no one else did anything
         about it. So, when it didn't occur that way, and the union office said to ring
         HR instead, it was full-on, full throttle. There was no misunderstanding
         that she was pissed off with me, but it was all that passive-aggressive bul-
         lying that if you didn't know, you wouldn't know.

Alex was in no doubt that the escalation in bullying behaviours was punishment
after she had publicly given evidence about bullying within the organisation:

> I testified before Parliament. I said things that were very uncomfortable for them to hear,
> and they never wanted anyone to hear. They're going to punish me for that. They're trying
> to make an example of me.

When Chris spoke out about her concerns and was no longer seen to support the
bully, she was treated entirely differently to other staff and singled out for
punishment:

> She'd put other people in the office I had been using and moved me into what could be
> described as a cupboard. One of the things that she expressed annoyance about was that I
> was the only one questioning the rationale behind the moves. I said, "I'm sorry that you're
> upset by me questioning that, but you'd given us the reasoning that you want people in
> teams to be in the same office. Based on that, I should be in this office over here. But you
> haven't done that, so I was just wondering why". And of course, I'd been isolated. That's
> how it felt. Other staff said, "It's very clear your move was a form of punishment".

Terry believed he was punished for whistleblowing when he discovered and
reported some funding anomalies that impacted his role:

He was instrumental in setting up the position I sit in. They were ripping off the donor organisation that I work with. So when I flagged that in the system and the ripping off had to stop, he got really pissed off with me, and I think I'm being punished for not supporting their greedy approach to this type of work.

7.8   Gender

I run into trouble because I'm a male in a female-dominated world. Sometimes I speak up when there's an expectation that I shouldn't be speaking up (Terry).

Shannon and Jesse saw gender as a significant factor in the bullying they experienced. They described a "boys' club" culture where successful women in senior positions upset the male-dominated status quo:

Shannon: I was the senior nurse. I was the only female at that time who was senior anything in the boys' club. So, I really think it was gender-based. I had been there for a long time and then got this opportunity, putting a lot of the boys' noses out. It was well known it was a boys' club, and no one was willing to call anyone on it.

Jesse: In my experience of academia, certainly, but also health services, if you're a woman, you really have to be much, much better than men. You really have to be remarkably better than men. I was developing an international reputation. My manager wasn't interested because, again, it was threatening. And you can't do much about that, young men being threatened by women of some solidity.

Terry believed that being male in nursing had been a contributing factor to being bullied by a female unit manager:

I run into trouble because I'm a male in a female-dominated world. Sometimes I speak up when there's an expectation that I shouldn't be speaking up, which got me into trouble with my manager.

7.9   Mental Health

As soon as stuff started going wrong and I started saying this was unfair, they started focusing more on mental health rather than what was actually going on (Rory).

Rory had a history of depression. She had told her mentor, believing she could trust her. Initially, she felt supported. However, once the bullying began, her mental health issues became a primary focus and a convenient diversion:

I had severe depression and had actually made a suicide attempt several months before I started working there. When I moved here, I'd found a GP and a psychiatrist. I was on medication, and I was trying to make things work. I didn't want to have any issues. After the emergency consultant returned from leave and the conversation started about the rotations, I told my mentor about my history. She felt she needed to tell the director of the department.

I'd met with both, and they said, "Listen, we just want to support you". I thought that was going to be the end of it. I thought everything was fine. But, as soon as stuff started going wrong and I started saying this was unfair, they started focussing more on mental health rather than what was actually going on. I just wanted transparency and answers. It was becoming extreme, and the bullying made me really suicidal again. My mentor had asked me whether I was having suicidal thoughts. I hadn't lied to her. I said yes, and then it all became about my mental health rather than dealing with the actual issue. I got frustrated by that. They made me get clearance to work, even though I was working in a new department, and they had no concerns about how I was functioning. Yeah. I felt like they were using it.

7.10 Personality

I don't have a problem if people don't like me … What bothers me is when people treat you differently depending on whether they like you (Jordan).

"If you're liked, you're fine. If you're not watch out", explained bullying for some champions. Taylor and Jordan were bullied many times because of personality issues rather than the issue or task at hand:

Taylor: They see the personality rather than the issue. If somebody does something good, I'll tell them I love what they have done and may even tell them I love them for doing it. But if they do something that isn't good for our community, I'll tell them. There can be people that I really despise how they've always worked. But if they do make a change for the better, I value them for making that change. That it's wonderful, I'm so proud of them. I can disassociate the past feelings for the person and their behaviour by appreciating the changes they are making now. I appreciate the strength and preparedness it takes to change what they have held onto for a long time.

Jordan: Sadly, many people can't keep personality or friendship out of professional and collegial relationships. I think of a colleague I worked with for a time. She was incredibly supportive of me and publicly praised me for my achievements. Unfortunately, it came to pass that we had a falling out for reasons I can only guess at, and her response to me since then couldn't be more opposite. We sat on a committee, and she challenged me on almost everything. I'm happy to be challenged on anything with a reasoned argument. These were not reasoned arguments. They were attacks. She would say dismissive, condescending, hostile and sometimes downright offensive things to me in front of others. As much as I was hurt and disappointed, I was intrigued. What thought processes go through someone's head when they react to people according to whether they like them or not? This was a woman with a senior position, highly experienced and had previously held managerial roles. Aside from being a health professional, couldn't she see that her responses were purely personal? My achievements and contributions hadn't changed because she no longer liked me. Couldn't she appreciate that whether you like someone should have no bearing on how you treat them professionally? I have seen it with so many people, yet I still find it beyond belief.

Sam was surprised that her senior manager saw the solution to her ongoing bullying as needing to "get on" with her senior nurse. Instead, Sam saw their professional relationship as the goal:

> "We have to find a way for you to get on". And I said, "Well, we don't have to get on. I don't understand what you mean. I don't have to be her best friend. I don't need new friends. We need to be able to work together in a professional capacity. She needs to acknowledge my existence. It's not about getting on".

These observations and other comments from the champions were particularly interesting. Like Sam, I don't need to be friends with people I work with, I don't need to like them, and I don't need them to like me. Unlike Sam, Taylor described herself as needing to be valued, respected, and liked, which had proved particularly challenging when working with people who clearly did not like her:

> I'm a person that likes to be valued, respected, and liked. And I hated that they didn't like me, you know? And I probably need to feel this way more than your average person, so it was really hard for me.

These comments prompted me to ask champions whether they needed to be liked. Sam, Jordan, Shannon, and Rory described themselves as emphatic but not needing to be liked. It was much more important to be valued and respected and to have open communication:

Sam: I don't care if you don't like me. I do mind if you don't respect me because I think like, and respect are different things. Staff can tell me, "Sam, I'm really pissed with you at the moment", and I say, "Why are you pissed with me? Let's talk about it".

Jordan: I don't have a problem if people don't like me. Some will, and some won't. I wouldn't have a problem if a colleague, manager, or whoever told me they didn't like me. I'd probably say, "Okay, thanks for your honesty, and that's no problem. I hope we can find a way to work together that acknowledges our contribution and the value we both bring". What bothers me is when people treat you differently depending on whether they like you.

Shannon: I don't need to be liked. I try to come across as someone who's engaging, helpful, and supportive, and if that's not good enough or if that's not what someone wants from me, then I don't know. So, no, I don't need to be.

Rory: I don't need to be liked. I just need to be treated with respect and fairness. I don't like everyone. I don't truly dislike that many people, but I definitely don't need to be liked myself.

Pat, Andy, and Jesse also didn't feel a strong need to be liked, although they did enjoy the opportunity to interact with colleagues and feel supported by them:

Pat: Not really. I'm there to do a job, not to make friends. It's good if f I've got someone I can sit and talk to at lunchtime because there are so many times I sit on my own. It's nice if you can sit and have some banter.

Andy: Less important, for sure, but it's good to have people you get along with and people you like because you spend a lot of time at work. So, it's nice to have some support, but I don't care about the people that don't care about me.

Jesse: I'd like to get on with everybody because I've always been a workaholic. Most of my socialising is with my work colleagues. So, I always want to get along with people, chat about things, have a pleasant relationship, and not have stress at work. I am happy with people who like to work hard and bounce ideas off. I work in teams. So, if I don't have a strong supportive team, I suffer because I've got to ask someone else: "I'm thinking this. What do you reckon?"

Terry and Chris initially said being liked was important to them. However, as our conversation progressed, it seemed that collegiality, acceptance, and respect were what they sought, and being liked was more a bonus than a necessity:

Terry: To me personally, it's very important. I'm not very comfortable in a workplace where I have to act differently from how I act outside of work, so being accepted for who I am is very important. My colleagues don't have to find me likeable. It's about accepting me as a person with all my strengths and flaws. Going out for an afternoon drink or coffee and spending the lunch break together chatting about life is important. I guess you like the people you do that with to a large extent. Fundamental respect for me as a person would be what I expect of others.

Chris: That's very important to me. I generally want my colleagues to be comfortable interacting and enjoy working and collaborating with me. In saying that, as I have gotten older, it's less impactful if they don't like me. When I was younger, I was like, "Oh my gosh" my self-esteem might have been more impacted. Now I can say, "Oh well, not everyone likes you and that's okay so long as you can still work effectively with people". Doing a good job is what trumps everything for me. I want to do a good job, and I want to be proud of the work that I do. I need to have effective work relationships to do that but that doesn't mean I have to be liked. There are lots of odd personalities that work in mental health, including myself. We tolerate the fact that we're all different and we're not all going to like everyone, and that's okay, but we've all got something to bring to the table. The diversity enriches the work that we do. I still think people need a sense of belonging, but you can belong without being liked so you can still feel connected to a team and have a purpose, even if you don't all want to hang out on the weekend. You can still respect each other and be inspired by each other even though you might say I disagree. I don't have to hang around with them as friends.

7.11   Being Me

> I've had periods when I thought I should keep my head down and not get involved in any-thing ... It's my personality to get involved, and I can't help it (Rory).

Champions displayed a strong and often irresistible desire to be themselves. They were very aware that changing their behaviour to be less assertive could have made their lives easier at work. However, they weren't willing to do so and believed this made them more likely to be bullied. Regardless, they were not willing to suc-cumb to expectations:

Rory: I've had periods when I thought I should keep my head down and not get involved in anything. But sometimes I can't help myself. I've managed to get involved in committees and writing proposals again, and having moments where I think, "Oh no, what if I step on people's toes?" It's my personality to get involved, and I can't help it.

Jesse: Unless you crawl up their bottoms and always tell them how great you are, you won't get anywhere, and I'm just not that person. A while ago, I asked: "What am I prepared to do to be successful? Am I going to lick arse?" No, I'm not, so I don't really care. I'm just not prepared to do that sort of soul-selling stuff that some people do, maybe, some people find it easy. That's not easy for me; no, I'm not going to. I work really hard, and I have the outcomes, the outputs. If you can't accept me for that, then I'm sorry, I can't do any more than that, and I'm not prepared to.

Jordan: I talked to my counsellor about my bullying experiences, and she said, "There's a pattern emerging here, isn't there?" So, we talked about that. I had thought before, is it me? Is there something I'm doing to make this happen? Something I can shut down to make this all go away? We talked about how I say what I think. I said, "That's how I am. I can't stand these people who walk around backslapping each other, pretending to be best friends, and would sell each other down the river if there was some advan-tage to be had. I'm not a sycophant, and I can't do that". She said that's fine. You need to keep in mind that your personality will attract bullies. It's obvious, but it was reassuring to know that I might not necessarily be able to stop this stuff from happening to me. But, at least I understood it and could make a choice. The choice to me was obvious. I refuse to be anyone other than me.

7.12   Basically, I Have No Idea

> The underlying question remains, why do people want to behave like that (Andy)?

Andy and Chris were at a loss in trying to understand why they had been targets. However, Andy remained curious, and Chris kept trying to convince herself about the real reason:

Andy: The underlying question remains, why do people want to behave like that?

Chris: There's a part of you that goes, why are you doing this to me? We have worked together for years, blah, blah, blah. But then there is this other part that goes, you know why she's doing this to you? Because she needs you gone, she needs to protect herself. You're trying to show others and make others aware of her behaviours.

With assistance from her psychiatrist, Alex realised that the problem lay with the bullies. Because they were so different in nature, she would likely never understand why they had chosen to bully her:

> I ask that question every day. The last time I talked to my psychiatrist, she said, "You're looking for an answer to a question that you're never going to get satisfied. There is a sociopath somewhere, and you can't reconcile what sociopaths do". She said, "You won't be able to understand this because you are such an empathetic person. You will have to start considering some of these people as a separate species because that's what they are. They don't care about how much they've harmed you; they actually delight in it. They don't have a conscience; they are not like you, so you've got to stop asking that question because the answer is there is no answer".

Life After Bullying

8

I'm not in any way ready to forgive these people, and I'm not ready to completely move on. I'm ready to move forward, but I'm not ready to be over it. I'm not there yet (Rory).

Workplace bullying is traumatic, and like all traumatic events, its effects can be felt long after it has ended. Some expect their lives to return to how they were before being bullied. They are often surprised when they still experience negative thoughts. Many targets seek advice on how to put these experiences behind them and return to their former selves.

An internet search of "how to recover or heal from workplace bullying?" reveals many resources from Australia and overseas. I once again had a strong sense of disappointment. Some constructive suggestions focused on health and self-care, seeking emotional support and staying connected with family and friends. I agree with the advice about not seeking revenge or publicly shaming the bully. Other suggestions sat much less comfortably with me. Don't dwell on the experience and avoid negative thoughts. If only it were that easy. Then we get to the stuff about moving on, closure and forgiveness. Sure, this would work for some, and that's great. Unfortunately, not everyone can move on or forgive that easily. Some champions were repeatedly bullied over long periods. Some have left jobs they loved and changed the course of their careers. This is much more than an unfortunate experience. They have suffered real loss and need to grieve. This must be acknowledged and respected, and targets should be supported rather than hit with platitudes. During our conversations, the champions talked about where they are now and how bullying has changed them.

B. Happell, *Sickness in Health: Bullying in Nursing and other Health Professions*, https://doi.org/10.1007/978-3-031-49336-2_8

8.1   Where Am I Now?

Some champions left jobs because of bullying, and some considered leaving. For some others, the bully was removed from the workplace; others still had ongoing issues.

Those Who Left

> It's been very, very disappointing. If I knew what I knew after two years in Australia, I would never have taken the job. I would have been in a more secure situation jobwise (Terry).

Champions who chose, or were strongly encouraged to, leave their workplace because of bullying and toxicity reflected on how they had changed. I have considered my own experiences a lot. I left more than one job because of bullying. After the last, I decided I would never work full-time again. Fortunately, I was of the age and financial status where that was an option. I now work part-time from home, and it's been fantastic in helping me settle into retirement. I love the work as I always have, and I don't have to deal with politics. Have I put the bullying behind me? Not completely. I sometimes still ask myself, "why did those bullies put so much time and effort into making it so hard for me to do my job?" It would help if I could understand it and give it some meaning. I know that will never happen. I don't see most of these people anymore, and I'm pretty sure they wouldn't take a call from me. Some would be surprised and possibly horrified that I considered them bullies. If they could be bothered thinking about it, they'd probably turn it back on me. Still, the questions go through my head, "why did you put so much effort into getting me to take that job and then put even more effort into making sure I couldn't do it properly?" I think about it less now. I'm sleeping better and having more fun. I expect it will always be there, though.

After being pressured to resign from her job for so long, Pat found a more flexible job, giving her greater scope to organise her working day. But, more importantly, she was able to enjoy her weekends again:

> We had a little afternoon tea here yesterday because it would have been my first son's 30th birthday had he lived. It was just nice to kick back and have a wine. It was good that I was able to enjoy myself. When everyone went, I sat down with a cup of coffee and thought okay, tomorrow's Monday. What have I got on? I checked my calendar. I've got a home visit, so I'll go into the office and then do that home visit. In the next couple of hours, our fridge died, so it was like, I'll go to the visit from home and spend the morning ringing for a repairman to fix the fridge. I managed to do that and did the visit.

When we spoke again about a year later, Pat had left that job because the role had become increasingly administrative, leaving less time with clients. She had recently started a job in a completely new area, and although faced with a steep learning curve, she felt supported:

I've been here for about six weeks. A bit out of my comfort zone because I haven't worked in this field. I'm learning new things. It is a supportive environment and very flexible. We've got to do on-call. I'm not so keen because I'm worried I will miss something because of my inexperience. My supervisor said, "don't worry about that because I'm your backup person. So, if you're not sure, just ring. We're a team. We help each other out."

Despite the more positive working environment, Pat still felt the effects of bullying. However, she now found herself better able to divert her attention than she had previously:

The sleep issues are still there. Sometimes it feels like I've still got an ear listening and aware of what's going on. I'm always tired when I wake up. Sometimes I wake up, and the first thing I think about is that place, weird. I can be in the car driving to work and replay something in my head. Now I say out loud, "no, stop, let it go," and then I can switch and think about something else. That helps.

Lee reflected on her decision to leave the workplace after her first bullying experience and its effect on the course of her career and that of many of her colleagues:

I was devastated because it was my area of expertise, and there weren't a lot of other places to go. Other places were also shedding workforce. Before I left, 30 other people had been cut by this woman. So, plenty of other people were in front of me in the queue. Some have done all sorts of different things. Some needed a couple of years off and therapy to get over it. Over time this woman had thwarted the career path of lots of us.

Jesse's career trajectory was also disrupted by bullying. She gave up a permanent position after a short secondment away from the bully because she couldn't bear to return to that environment. Now she was unemployed:

I'm currently unemployed. I would still have a job if he hadn't forced me out. I was in a permanent position at a nice wage, a mid-manager in a health service. I could've stayed there. It was a job for life, and I had to give that up. Given how hard I've worked all my life and how productive I've been, I'm guessing that I wouldn't really be semi-retired if I hadn't had the bullying. It had a substantial impact on my career path. I have suffered emotionally and have a lot of physical issues. I'm pretty relaxed about things, but I still sometimes think, what if? What might have been?

I asked Jesse if she were angry about how bullying had affected her career. Her opinion of the bullies had been a protective factor from anger, and overall, she was happy with her life:

I think those people are pathetic. I actually feel a bit sorry. This is how I cope with stuff. I'm not angry because I don't think people like that are in control of what they're doing. They're bound by quite narcissistic personalities. They don't have the Insight, don't have empathy, and I don't think they understand what they're doing. So, I don't have that many bad feelings about it. I'm happy where I am. My life has changed, but I'm in a good place.

When we last spoke, I asked Jesse if she still felt any impact from the bullying:

Every so often, I think about it and process it again. Honestly, I'm very much don't cry over spilt milk. Bridges have been crossed, and I don't like going backwards, and I don't like post-mortems very much, so I wouldn't talk to these people about it. I don't think about it often, but it does pop up if I feel down about what I am doing here.

Jordan ultimately made the decision to leave for the sake of her health and well-being:

I knew I needed to leave. The environment was not good for my health, and I knew it wouldn't get any better. I felt I'd done everything I could. It wasn't easy making that decision because I still thought I had so much to contribute. I did procrastinate for a while. My decision was made easier when the university offered voluntary separations. That gave me a finishing date. That was it. Time to retire. I wasn't going to start all over in a new job, a new location. It had exhausted me.

In our last conversation, Jordan described still feeling the effects of bullying several years after retiring:

I'm sad to say I still find myself ruminating about things that happened. It's been hard to cope with knowing all the work the team and I had put into getting this centre up and running, creating a national and international reputation, was for nothing. The centre continues in name, but the entire team I recruited is now gone and it is effectively dying a slow death. Not only is it personally disappointing, it is a wicked and immoral waste of public money. So yes, I still hold some anger and a whole of disappointment. It's becoming less and less. I still don't understand what motivates people to be bullies. I do understand it at an intellectual level but not an emotional one. Health professionals are supposed to care, not destroy the lives of people who want to make a difference.

Rory was awaiting a response to her official complaint to the health department. On advice, she sought documents through freedom of information from her former employee. However, after her requests were stalled several times, she was presented with incomplete information:

I filed an application for my HR file and emails or communications regarding me. It usually takes six weeks, and they asked for an extension. I granted the extension, and the day that I was meant to receive the information, I didn't hear anything. Because they missed the date, I could either start the process again or apply for an external review. I didn't trust the process and applied for an external review. Again, there were extension requests and failure to provide documents by the deadline. I eventually received 270 pages, most of it were documents I already had. An extraordinary amount was missing. I didn't learn anything more about why or who had done what they did. I then had to write a list of everything missing in as much detail as possible, going over everything again. They then went back to the hospital and requested more, but I'm still waiting. I think it's being intentionally dragged out, so I eventually give up.

I last spoke with Rory soon after she had received the outcome of her complaint. No fault was found, and no action would be taken against her former employers. She was understandably disappointed:

I was upset for a day or two, but I wasn't too dysfunctional. My thoughts were more that this was an unfair process rather than this is a reflection on me. I knew it was very likely that this was going to happen. I still feel disappointed. This was an opportunity for the Health Department to say, "here was an episode of serious bullying, and we've got a lot of evidence to support that." Instead, they chose to cover it up. They did admit that HR did not follow the correct processes but concluded there would have been no change to the outcome. I contest that. They've come to these conclusions because it's easier, and there's nothing I can do about it. It took 20 months in total for this process. Everyone kept warning me this might be the outcome. Still, I had this hope that maybe not, because I'd gone to the effort of getting the evidence, and maybe someone decent would be involved in the decision, but no.

I asked Rory: where to from here? Had she considered other avenues, or was it time to let the matter go? She was still considering options, although they didn't look very encouraging:

I've written to the health minister, asking for a review of this decision. I haven't received a reply yet. I did speak to a lawyer about my legal options. Because I returned to work after several months, I can't argue for lost income. Legally, it's all about money. He said there were really no legal options, and if I did try, it would cost me $50,000, with nothing to gain. He said the ombudsman is about making system changes, so they're unlikely to care much about individual bullying. There's the option of making individual complaints about specific clinicians to AHPRA (Australian Health Professionals Registration Authority). I'm also thinking about how my training college dealt with me. I've had zero communication from them, and they have expressed that they will support the hospital, not me. I'm also considering whether I go to the medical council and make a complaint once I'm in a less precarious position with my training.

We talked about how this latest development had affected her overall well-being, and thankfully the impact was not too extreme:

It's still something that's on my mind, but not all the time. But no, I don't think it's affected me any more than it already was. I guess I was just waiting, and waiting, and waiting for a response anyway.

On a more positive note, Rory's new job was completely different. She was highly regarded and had received unexpected and welcome recognition, an honourable mention for a well-being award:

I'm now in a very lovely workplace. It has reasonable leadership and good relationships between doctors and nurses. I don't know of any major bullying that's going on. I've had completely positive feedback. My assessments say, "she's an asset to the department," nothing negative. I won the registrar of the year award and this Well-being Award—twice now! It's an award where people nominate other people. I have absolutely no idea who nominated me or what it was for. It was so lovely.

After experiencing frequent bullying episodes in different workplaces, Taylor was now in a very positive environment where she felt respected and valued and had no fears of bullying. In fact, behaviours that might lead to bullying were addressed immediately:

It's very different working in the service I work for now and with the manager I have. One person tried to intimidate me. That was managed very well and very respectfully. However, the person who initiated the intimidation never fully accepted their behaviour. My CEO and the general manager of HR talked with me. They included my partner in the whole process and plan of management. They helped me understand the responses from the person as being self-preservation rather than trying to be hurtful. Because I can see and engage with the other's viewpoint, it's been healing. It has enabled the best relationships for the service and ourselves. We never really got to the bottom of it. They'd say things like "I'm sorry you felt that I was threatening," rather than "I'm sorry I did that." I find that pretty offensive. They're not holding themselves accountable. Still, my CEO and the HR manager helped me not to be overly affected or emotionally crippled by it. They made me feel they understood what had happened and how I felt.

Despite her more positive working environment, Taylor still found herself affected by bullying experiences from the past:

If I interact with those people, I still automatically feel intimidated and fearful. I also feel inadequate, that I haven't dealt with it and haven't the strength to not allow those people to affect me that way. I also feel that if I had been stronger, pushed the barrow, and made the services more accountable for what had happened, other people may not have been subject to the same behaviour.

In my last conversation with Terry, his contract had ended and had not been renewed. He had an extra year of work with the not-for-profit organisation. While he was enjoying this working environment, job insecurity was taking its toll. He was also dealing with the disappointment that the job had not been as he expected:

I should have been here five years ago because it's a good organisational fit. The only thing that puts me under pressure now is that I need the permanency of a position to plan anything. I feel paralysed because I can't really plan. The contract will continue for a year, and if I can't find a job in Australia within that time, that's the end of me in Australia. If I'm on short-term contracts, I can't be the researcher I want to be. It's been very, very disappointing. If I had known what I knew after two years in Australia, I would never have taken the job. I would have been in a more secure situation jobwise.

Terry talked about the ongoing impacts of bullying now he had left the health service:

I think I feel better. My blood pressure is slightly high. I think it's related to that type of stress. I struggle with interpersonal stress, and not having to be confronted with that on a weekly basis is a huge relief. I feel I'm recovering and can focus on getting a new job. I still have nightmares. I'm haunted by the two bullies in my dreams. I was going to a conference recently, but I knew he would be there, so I didn't. It feels like a relationship breakup where I am fearful of meeting my former partner. I'm upset about it, I wish I could repair it, but I don't see it's an option. Usually, I'm successful in what I do in my work life, so there's a strong sense of failure. I didn't want the relationship. I found it violent, and I didn't thrive in it. At the same time, I feel like I failed in managing the relationship. I'm scared of applying for jobs where I know the bully would have an influence.

Those Champions Considering Leaving

> I would feel so anxious to see either of those girls again. I would avoid it like the plague. I get triggered by the little thing from teams. This is a message. Shit, what's it going to say? (Shannon).

Champions who remained in the job where the bullying continued were contemplating leaving. However, Lee was feeling ambivalent about making that decision:

> I'm finishing things off and getting myself into a state of preparedness. I'll have a trained team. This is done, that's done, the ship won't sink. I don't know why I should care about a ship that hasn't done anything for me. That's about the common good, not about you, but at least I'll have a chance to think. And then, the thought of going to another job and learning, da-da-da-da, it's overwhelming.

After making the decision to leave, Shannon was offered a new job quite out of the blue:

> It's with someone that I've worked with off and on for about 20 years. I saw her about some of her clinical incidents and spoke to them about clinical governance and risk. And she just said, "Oh my God, we need you here." And I went, "Really?" She said, "What's your dream job look like?" I went, "A little bit of clinical, a little bit of supervision, a little bit of leadership. I'll do some clinical governance, risk management, and quality." And she said, "All right." I wasn't going for a job interview. I was going to slap them on the wrist for not performing to standards. And I walk out with a job. They 100% listened to my areas of interest and expertise. I can't believe it. I'm actually feeling wanted. And that has given me a boost to my confidence. I feel I'll be supported in this role because they want it to work so much.

Despite her experiences of bullying and lack of support, Shannon still felt some guilt about leaving her current job:

> I think I'll hold guilt because I feel like I've let the organisation down, particularly my line manager. We're already two staff down, and we're going to be three, potentially four. And she's still going to be there. That lady needs a lot more support than she's getting. I haven't left previously because of her. I was honest with the new place that we had a huge transition to get through, and I would only be willing to leave after that work is done, as I feel obliged.

By our last conversation, Shannon had commenced her new job. She was enthusiastic about the workplace and her role:

> It's a really positive environment. Management really looks after you. Even though we're not doing Covid anymore, they still allow us to work at home. It's nice to be able to support people to do that.

Shannon's decision to leave her previous workplace was made easier by the Covid pandemic that brought the bullying into her own home:

> I was hanging on by my fingernails, and my fingernails just broke. The straw that broke the camel's back was bullying coming through into my home life and my house, on the phone, on speaker or teams messages that would pop up on the screen. Constantly put down. The

way I work is you always give good feedback. If you have to give bad feedback, you put it in a feedback sandwich. You always pump people's tyres up as best you can, and mine kept getting let down and let down. You fucked up again. There is no way I would ever speak to anyone like that.

I asked Shannon about the response to her resignation:

It didn't go down very well. The general manager asked me to withdraw my resignation because she felt she could fix things. I think they understood because they ended up making the bully staff redundant. I had an interview with the general manager and the service development manager. I expressed my concerns to them. I was very clear about what the problem was.

Shannon talked about the residual effects of her recent bullying that still lingered:

I would feel so anxious to see either of those girls again. I would avoid it like the plague. I get triggered by the little thing from teams. This is a message. Shit, what's it going to say? If the people's names that come up are people I worked with in that organisation, it just brings me straight back. I don't dream about it. It's going to take its natural course, and I know in time I'll hear that ding and think it's a doorbell.

Those Where the Bully Was Removed

Even if I left tomorrow, I would need two or three months off to recover from this. It feels so draining. I wouldn't want to go on holidays because I'd feel like I would take this with me (Lee).

Chris felt enormous relief after the bully was removed. However, she was disappointed by the lack of support and debriefing, particularly given what the organisation stood for:

Once you're out of the situation, there's that initial relief. Thank goodness, I don't actually have to face this person again. I can now focus on trying to recover from a traumatic experience. This massive weight is lifted off your shoulders. That was a fabulous outcome. Now, the details of the ins and outs, don't know, not privy to. There wasn't an official statement to say that the behaviours have been really bad, and that's why this person's no longer here, probably for legal reasons. There hasn't been any opportunity to bring staff together to work out; how do we move on from this? How do we make sure this never happens again? If you don't ever do those restorative practices, it is hard for people to have closure and to move on.

Chris was feeling more positive during our last conversation. However, healing from the trauma was a work in progress, and she could still be triggered 2 years later:

I definitely have some residual stuff. I think the basic things have healed. My sleep is not impacted anymore, and I don't experience anxiety. When you have these experiences, you still carry them with you at times. Just when you think you've left it behind, something happens, and you're brought right back there again. Last week I had to facilitate training with someone who had witnessed the workplace bullying towards me and supported the bully. When I was told I needed to conduct training with this person, I could feel the same physical sensations, the butterflies. The fight/flight response is triggered, and you're immediately taken back to a time when you didn't feel safe. I'm thinking, "I can't believe I have to be in the room with this person for 4 days." I managed very well. I made sure I wasn't asking too much of myself and had good self-care. My mantra was, "just do your best and be your friendly, warm, competent professional self." It was a big week, but we got through. It never ceases to amaze me, the bullying experience was two years ago, and 99% of the time, you don't think about it, have processed it. Then it doesn't take much for you to go right back there again. When you have these experiences, there are times when you have to watch yourself: "am I moving into an automatic assumption that the same things are going to happen again?" When you're interacting with people with these established patterns of behaviour, you also think it could happen. It has happened in the past.

Chris was disappointed that most of her colleagues did not express concern or offer support to her for having to work with this person:

Someone said, "this week could be difficult for Chris," but nobody picked up the phone and asked how are you doing with that? And thank you for doing that. One of the frustrating parts of this organisation is how bad they are at this stuff, and I don't know why. I'm so shocked they cannot practice what they preach. It's hard for me to get my head around. They know what the research says, and they're so bad at dealing with conflict within the organisation.

Chris remained concerned about her reputation. She was unsure of how others saw her and the role she may have played in having the bully removed:

"What is their opinion of me?" Even though I can say to myself, "Yeah, yeah," I was appropriate and professional and didn't do anything I can't stand by. But you're left going, "Yeah, but did the bully leave enough doubt in other people's minds about me?" Sometimes I think there are people I had really good working relationships with before, and the relationship is different now. So you think: "Is there doubt in their mind about me because of what the bully was saying and doing?" Who knows?

After the initial relief, Lee found herself exhausted and still strongly impacted by her experiences:

Even if I left tomorrow, I would need two or three months off to recover from this. It feels so draining. I wouldn't want to go on holidays because I'd feel like I would take this with me. I'm still a bit in a doghouse, "you went to the Board. Maybe you can't be trusted." It's like, "Are you fucking serious? Twelve people left. This is not in my imagination. The Board sacked her." Twenty-two people spoke to the lawyer. Before the investigation was even half over, they'd stood her down and locked her out of the building. As she was leaving, she made out that I was difficult and wasn't getting things done. Despite the fact none of that was true, it is very hard to go back to people and say, "I don't know what she told you, what you think I did and what you heard from her because you're not telling me." Some things I have heard or worked out, I could say, "Here's the email. That's not true. Why would you believe this psychopath when you know she's a raging bully? Yet you've chosen to believe some of the things she's said."

Lee's actions had been instrumental in the bully's departure. However, she was disappointed by the lack of acknowledgement. Lack of attention to the mental health and well-being of those people who had been adversely affected by the bullying persisted despite promises this would be addressed:

I've gone from being very kindly disposed towards the organisation and the Board. I feel like I saved them because everyone else was terrified, but I went, "No, I've seen this before." I put my big girl pants on, wrote to them, and put it on the record so they could save the organisation and get rid of this woman. Not one of them has thanked me, and not one of them has done anything. In my document, I'm saying, "These are the things that my colleagues have reported: no sleep, anxiety, stress, crying." Nobody came to me in the intervening nine months and said, "How're you going?" We only got a generic "there's employee assistance program if you want it." We asked many times what had happened. "Can you just give us, if you don't want it in writing, just a little general talk?" We put in all the effort we had to suffer from this woman and helped get rid of her and all her cronies. We all fucking knew she was running the place down and putting us at huge reputational risk. Nothing. They said they would set up a well-being committee and train people, but most people who were impacted got nothing. The woman who interviewed us for that report said she would recommend training for the Board, all of us, supportive things, to help us coalesce and come together afterwards. Nothing happened. Often these psychopaths split the team, and she did that very effectively, and it hasn't come back together.

The lack of consequences for the bully also made it quite possible her behaviour would move on rather than be addressed:

What often happens in these places is the lawyers get in between. I'm sure that's what happened at our place. They cancel their contracts and agree to no disparagement, but there's no record or trace of these people. That's why I make the analogy to the Pell priests. They just turn up somewhere else.

In our last conversation, I asked Lee how she found the environment now. She was clearly still impacted and was disappointed in herself for feeling this way:

Some parts of it are better, but there are legacies from the past. We're a divided camp. Some new people don't know anything, older people who were allies of the CEO and her bully friends and a small group of people who stood up to them. Some didn't ally themselves but were witnesses and didn't do anything. I'm even more annoyed now. At the time, I was so tired and beleaguered by it. I'm still mad at myself, wishing I'd done what I would have told someone else to do, stand back, get the lawyers in, get the union. I'm annoyed that I didn't just nip it in the bud and stand up for myself. They pushed her out, but they've done nothing for us. Their response is really pathetic, given the space we are in. I still think about it more than I'd like to. A lot of the time, you're okay. But, every now and again, you come up against something in the workplace and go, "you've been incredibly difficult about this," and how safe and comfortable they feel in behaving in really appalling ways.

She gave an example of how a simple request to purchase masks made to a former ally of the bully played out and impacted her:

I wrote to her and said can you get me a quote for some masks, and it just cracked on from there. "Have you thought about this? have you thought about that? I'm thinking with my occupational health and safety hat." It went on and on. I said, "Thanks, yes, we know how to do this safely." She wrote back again, and this went on for half the week. She had a meeting with the head of finance, and I'm like, "why? you were just asked to get a quote for some masks." In the end, I copied in the CEO to show her what I had to deal with. She sent me some quotes and details of places I had asked her not to get quotes from. "I can just be difficult because we were in this little game, and we got away with it." There was still no penalty for her taking a whole week to get masks. In the end, I got them myself, which I could have done in 10 minutes, but I was directed to ask her. If I have to do something involving about a third of the staff, I have to think about it in detail, so no one could mis-construe anything. The CEO sees it and is outraged but doesn't do anything about it. It's exhausting.

When the bully was dismissed from Andy's workplace, there was a major upheaval, leaving the remaining staff short of skilled people for the job:

She was asked to leave in the end. Staff were thankful, "Okay, we'll just take a breath because this has been out of control for some time." It was a tough time because quite a few staff left. It was horrendous for those of us left because we were left with the fallout and no staff. It's been a constant rebuild from when she left. She tried to destroy the department. She tried to get us all to leave and get a job at her new place. "Why would I want to go and work for you when I know what you're like?" It was about her sticking it up the hospital. She was trying to decimate the service, sticking the knife into them because they told her to pack her bags and go.

Although she was no longer bullied, Andy did not believe the workplace had recovered since the bully left. Her attitude to work had changed significantly:

We have an environment that's quite divided. Over the years, it's gotten more and more and more. We were a very close-knit tight team. I do my job to the best of my ability, but I'm not doing anything extra. I'm not doing work at home. It's turned people to feel that way. The boss does nothing to bring the team together.

The bullying experiences made Andy warier and less likely to stick her neck out with her concerns or opinions:

Every now and again, something will happen that will cause me to reflect on what might be going on in the environment. Is this going to lead to something else? It makes you a little gun-shy. If that situation hadn't happened, you'd probably be freer to say, think, or do. I still say what I think, just a little gun-shy about saying too much because you never know where something will go, even when you feel you've done everything right. I certainly didn't think I'd done anything that deserved the reactions and responses from this person, and I don't want to experience that sort of shit again.

8.2   Those Still Dealing with Bullies

I don't know if I'll ever be employable again. I don't even know if I'll ever be able to leave my house and feel safe again. It's been horrific (Alex).

During our conversations, Alex was on WorkCover and trying to reach a resolu-tion with her employer. Unfortunately, the impact of the bullying and the prolonged resolution process has left her exhausted, frustrated and, at times, suicidal:

It's a daily battle for my sanity, for my health, and it's ruined my and my husband's dreams here. Our entire life has been shattered. I don't know where I'm going after this. I don't know if I'll ever be employable again. I don't know if I'll ever be able to leave my house and feel safe again. It's been horrific, and the member of parliament who actually gave me a slot to testify, I reached out to his office. I was not in a good place. I was suicidal, and I wrote him an incredibly emotive letter. I told him what had happened to me. Since I testified, this is the retaliation that I'm facing. Because of COVID-19, I'm now being told it will be two-and-a-half to three years before the court hears my case. So, I will have to try to hang on to any sanity I might have until then. He wrote back, "Is it okay if I confidentially reach out to the minister and the commissioner? I'm quite concerned about some of the things you've told me." I said, "It doesn't have to be confidential at this stage. I do not care anymore. I feel like I'm in an abusive domestic relationship with them that I cannot get divorced from, and I just want the divorce final."

When last we spoke, some 10 months later, Alex had not heard from the politician, which she seemed to accept with quiet resignation after so many avenues of potential help had come to nothing. Her court hearing was expected up to 10 months away. The toll it was taking on her health and well-being was extreme:

I am in therapy right now. I had to go to court to win the battle for that treatment. I'm very deflated and very defeated. Sometimes I sit here and think I just want to get out of this situation alive. It's very suffocating. I don't have any support. My family is not here. My friends aren't here. It's a suffocating feeling. You don't know what's coming around the next corner. It's terrifying. It's like you're on a ride, you can't get off. In normal life, when you're in a distressing circumstance, you can leave and have enough control to plan your way out. I can't do that here. I'm stuck in this for as long as I'm stuck in it.

The bullying continued for Alex as she moved closer to her case being heard. She was hesitant to leave the house alone. She feared management of the organisation was watching and monitoring her and attempting to control her access to medication:

I'm very hesitant about going out because it's winding down towards the end of my case. I'm concerned about what surveillance they would be doing and the extremes they may go to. They make me feel unsafe, and I know they're watching my attendance at therapy because the girls at the front desk gave me the heads-up. I feel like a prisoner. It'll be five years in May, and that's a long time not to have control over your life. So, I'll only leave if I have someone with me. I usually take Valium before I go out because I get so panicked. The ambulance service has made it very difficult for me to get the medication I need. They made a veiled accusation that I was abusing drugs. They sent letters to all my doctors asking about my medications. So, my doctor has become very cagey about prescribing it for me.

At her lowest point, Alex was suicidal and entirely dependent on her family. She believed some responses from the Ambulance service were deliberately intended to encourage her to take her own life:

I had become so unwell. My husband couldn't work in shifts, and my son had to cut his work schedule back because they were scared to leave me alone. I got to the point where I told them very graphically that I wanted to kill myself. I believe that was why the ambulance service stopped the therapy and tried to get some of my medication removed, hoping I would commit suicide. I think they were trying to push me over the edge.

Alex also believed the organisation was trying to break her financially with additional legal costs:

A hundred and twenty thousand so far. It's had a huge impact, we used to have a great life-style, and now we are on a shoestring budget to pay the legal costs, which will only increase. If we do recover anything financially, a lot will go on legal bills. It scares me what is going to happen to us. They asked for my passport, bank records and tax returns for the last six years. The solicitor said they don't really have a valid reason. They are doing this to harass you and have you send all these documents that will increase your legal bill.

Alex described herself as absolutely dispirited and deflated by her protracted experiences. Not surprisingly, her self-care had taken a beating. She wished she had never set foot in the Ambulance Service:

I haven't been taking care of myself. I started having difficulty walking and didn't know what was wrong with me, but I tore some tendons. I'm 41 years old, but I probably have the physical fitness of somebody in their 70s. I don't sleep very well. I get panicked. If I have a nightmare or there's a noise that wakes me, I can't go back to sleep. I wasn't eating. Now I have a meal delivery service, so I try to have at least one meal a day that is nutritious and balanced. I am making small steps, but my life is still extremely abnormal. I wish I could hit the rewind button. If I knew then what I know now, I would have walked out after that assault and never gone back. It's horrific that you go to work to do your job, get injured and then you're brutalised for it. Reporting it becomes the offence.

When we last spoke, Sam had recently learned that her request to reclassify her position had been denied. Her frustration was only surpassed by her determination to see the reclassification succeed:

It's very hard. Even the union have not been very proactive. I have to continually ring and say where are we up to? The union wrote to the director of nursing asking when the reclas-sification meeting is. She wrote back and said they had met. They didn't include the union in the correspondence, nor me. I wrote to her requesting a meeting. The union says they don't know how things would go if we went to Fair Work Australia. They have suggested we go for the difference in money. The difference is negligible. I have never been interested in the money. I've been interested in recognition for the role, particularly a career pathway for nurses. It's not about me. How do I make this a job that anyone would want to touch? It's been nearly two years. I hoped to get the classification sorted out before putting bullying on the table. I don't want the two to be connected. Sam continued to be ignored by her senior nurse and was not provided with critical information that she needed for her job:

One of my wards is undergoing significant stress. I'm considerable staff down with the greatest demand for these services in 30 years. The state senior nurse advisor sent an email to the senior nurse. Saying she would like to meet with her and me to discuss the stress being felt by the nurses. This is not communicated to me by the senior nurse and still has not been. She sent everyone else the email but not me.

Sam was still feeling the ongoing impacts of the bullying, particularly affecting her sleep:

I still have trouble sleeping. If something is coming up or I've read something, I get angry and can't sleep. I'm worried about the upcoming meeting about my role. It's always there beneath the surface.

8.3   Me After Bullying

> Some of my views and attitudes have changed a little, but fundamentally no, I don't think
> I've changed. I still have the same principles about how to treat people (Jordan).

Throughout our conversations, the champions would talk about how bullying had changed them, particularly their relationships with colleagues and attitude towards bullying. During our last conversation, I asked all champions this question. Jesse talked about her changed career trajectory and the disappointment she still carried with her:

> I have a changed trajectory. I don't get angry or hurt, just disappointed. There's this emo-
> tional baggage I had to work on to get rid of. I'm definitely a changed person.

Alex described herself as virtually unrecognisable from the person she was before her bullying experiences:

> I will never be the same, and I feel really conflicted. I don't know if I'll ever feel like a
> normal human being. It's definitely changed my perception of Australia. I hate that because
> I wanted to live my whole life here. I feel like I'm surrounded by people who hate my very
> existence. I'm stuck. I don't know if I can ever fix it. That's the scariest part.

Rory considered herself both changed and the same person. It was quite enlightening to listen to her work through this dilemma:

> I think I'm a changed person and the same person. I view the hospital system very differ-
> ently. I'm a lot warier of people. That doesn't come across in day-to-day circumstances, but
> I'm much more aware of people in power. So, I have this sense that I'm the same person I
> was, yet I've had these wildly different experiences. So, I'm certainly different in some
> regards.

Lee considered herself a changed person. This was really obvious at work and had encroached on her personal life to some degree:

> Yes, I am I don't think I would have wanted to admit that a year or two ago. I'm more cau-
> tious because I become like, "what's she up to? What's happening here?" I'm more hyper-
> vigilant, even if people don't warrant it all the time. I'm also bolder. I think fuck you, I'm
> not putting up with that, whereas before I let a few things go through to the keeper, now I'm
> just going to stand up and nip that in the bud. Sometimes, I've been less social because I've
> been exhausted from overthinking and protecting myself.

Sam was also warier of colleagues and was less likely to promote her own contributions to the service because she feared the repercussions:

> It's probably made me very wary about who I trust. I'm less likely to put myself out there
> in areas where I could have my service excelling. I've had a couple of publications and
> international conference presentations. I haven't sent that to the heads. I don't want to put
> myself out there to be criticised.

Chris talked about the ways bullying had changed her as a person. While most were negative, she also identified some positives:

> Definitely, I'm much warier. I don't automatically assume that people are out to get me. I'm realistic that there really are people in the world who harm people and are okay with that. That makes me a changed person because I was much more trusting early on. I'm such an open book, upfront and direct. I took everyone at face value, and with my many experiences, I now realise that you can't do that. People will say one thing to your face and do something very differently behind your back. Do I feel anxiety more than I used to, or am I just more aware that it does happen? Observe it in my body more? Maybe part of me feels stronger. I'm more resilient in some ways. If I found myself there again, this is what I would do, and this is how I would handle it. So, you feel like you've grown from the experience and learnt stuff. It's not all bad. You'd prefer not to have the experience.

Chris had also used her first two experiences as learning which had helped her feel the bullying less at a personal level:

> By this third time, because I've had these experiences and know what these behaviours are, there wasn't the self-doubt or not to the same extent. I was much more matter of fact, this is what's happening, and this is what I can do. I didn't feel the same powerlessness that only came from reflecting on that second experience.

Andy noted the changes to her as a person in both her professional and personal life:

> I take a step back a little to review, where I would blindly assume everything was okay. I'm more of an advocate for others to document and look at what's happening. This is not appropriate. Let's try to nip it in the bud. It's made me stick up a bit more during Covid. I eliminated people from my life because they bullied me on Facebook. I do not need this. Enough is going on without this aggravation. Fuck it. I'm not putting up with it.

Terry considered himself a changed person in some ways, and yet still felt fundamentally the same:

> I think I'm a changed person in the sense of feeling like a failure. It will be an experience that I take with me, a bit like a battle scar, it won't fundamentally have changed me, but it's on me. Some days I will be able to see it but not think about it all the time as I did when it happened. The thing that will be interesting for me is if I experience something similar again, how will I be re-traumatised? How will old feelings come back, and with what force? I think my drive into the world is the same. I've got a scar I will wear forever. I would be triggered by others being bullied, but I don't know if the trigger would paralyse me or start some kind of protective manoeuvre. I've got more respect for the impact of bullying. The good thing is I don't see it every day in the workplace I'm in right now.

Jordan did not believe she had fundamentally changed as a person at all:

> Some of my views and attitudes have changed a little, but fundamentally no, I don't think I've changed. I still have the same principles about how to treat people with fairness and justice, honesty and openness. If I started another job, I would be much more careful with managers, bystanders and hecklers. I know I will always carry this with me. At times I wish I didn't have to. Other times it's important to hold onto these experiences and use them in a

way that helps break down this hideous bullying problem that we have in health. I have supported people being bullied. It has taken a while to heal, but I'll come out with something to offer. I am still fundamentally a decent human being.

8.4   Changing How I Relate to Colleagues

There are people I won't talk to and associate with because I know people who work there do not have my back … It absolutely makes you not talk or relate to people the same way (Andy).

In the *chapter what bullying did to me,* the champions discussed the loss of friendships and collegial relationships and the distress this caused them. More than that, these broken relationships fundamentally changed some champions, leaving them wary and guarded. For example, Jesse became both less trusting and less tolerant:

I take everything with a grain of salt. "That might be true. It might not." I've got a fairly thick skin, so I try not to let stuff get to me. I've got a true understanding that this is all about them and not me. I still interact with many colleagues, but I won't put up with any bullshit. If I have to deal with someone I don't like, I walk away. I can pick someone who's going to be a problem quickly, and I go, no, I'm not interacting with this person. It's not worth my while. You can't pay me that much.

Chris and Lee had lost trust in their colleagues through their ordeals. As a result, they had become more vigilant, carefully collecting evidence for anything that might become a bone of contention in the future:

Chris: I'm way less trusting than I used to be. I think more about ensuring that if something was to ever come back on me, I've got evidence. I wouldn't say I assume that people don't have the right motives or intentions. I don't. I generally take people at face value, but I always have in the back of my mind that you have to protect yourself. You can't just automatically trust everyone. If it's not in writing, you've got nothing to fall back on. I trust my instincts and intuition more than I did years ago and am confident to say I won't put myself in that position. Years ago, I probably would think it was all in my head.

Lee: I'm pretty careful about putting things in writing or on Skype. I see something from them that I'm not sure of, I take a screenshot. When all the trouble happened, and people tried to report me, I had records. If somebody does terrible things, I send it straight to my director and say: I've told you about issue x, and any time I see an example of issue x I'm sending it on to you. So later on, if they don't do anything or something comes up, I first alerted them in June 2020 and sent 20 examples of this behaviour. If they choose not to act on it, something happens. Well, I'm completely covered.

Andy's experiences made her much more cautious about what she said to managers and colleagues:

The bottom line for me is that everyone should be treated fairly and equally; obviously, that doesn't happen. You might think you're being treated fairly for a while, but then you realise you're not. It changes your perspective on the next manager. You're not going to say things you might have said before, like when I explained to my manager that she didn't take my job. If I said nothing, I'm in trouble. If I say something, I'm in trouble, so I may as well say nothing. I will hold my cards close to my chest a bit more. Even currently, there are people I won't talk to and associate with because I know they do not have my back. They are out to take you by the knees as quickly as they can. It absolutely makes you not talk or relate to people the same way.

Rory found herself reflecting more about her own communication and trying to demonstrate the kind of behaviour she thought was appropriate in the workplace:

I'm much more aware that the little comments can be really damaging. When I see someone being snappy, they may be exhausted or in a not-quite-right frame of mind. If I can, I'll make a joke, or take them aside and say, "are you okay with that? That was really out of line." I'm more aware of what's going on and just trying to model how we should treat each other.

When Shannon commenced her new job, previous experiences made her aware of what she needed from the organisation. Now she had the confidence to ensure she received it:

I'm going in as a manager with that mindset. Not to control, but to be confident that I trust the organisation to train me properly, so I am informed and can do my job well. I have spoken to them very discretely and professionally. One of my clear expectations is that my orientation is worthwhile and useful. Because my orientation at the last job was not, that is a big fear of mine, and I feel they will take that on.

I've certainly had my fair share of friends or people I considered friends who betrayed me. Some barely would acknowledge my existence when I was no longer of use to them. I remind myself of the friends I met through work who are still part of my life. I have some beautiful friends I met through work. If I had allowed past experiences to completely destroy my trust in colleagues, they would not be the important part of my life that they are now. I refuse to let those poisonous and self-interested so-called friends or colleagues affect me any more than they already have. I'm sad and a little regretful, but I'm not willing to let their nastiness change how I relate to others. Managers are a different story. I would be much more careful about setting clear expectations with managers. I'd want agreement about what they want from me, what resources are available, and, most importantly, how we would deal with emerging issues. I would have it all in writing. I know that's not foolproof. One boss would dispute what we had previously agreed to. Then, when I showed her the email chain, she would change the tone and say, "Well, I don't have any budget for it," and tell me how lucky I was with what I already had. I would protect myself as much as possible, and I would also be well aware of the fact that even that may not be enough.

8.5   Views About Bullying

> I was a person who stood up for others more than I will now. If I stick up for you, you'll leave me in the lurch, and I'm going to sink, and I can't be bothered with it (Jesse).

Rory believed her own experiences had made her unwilling to tolerate others being bullied:

> A consultant was bullying one of the other registrars, whom he perceived as weak. They weren't weak. They were not as experienced. I was angry about how he treated her when it was meant to be his job to support her. A lot of that came from what had happened to me.

Chris was insistent she was now unwilling to work in an organisation that allowed bullying to continue:

> It comes down to the organisation. If it doesn't have the same values as me or can't live by them, do I want to continue working there? Five or six years ago, this wouldn't have been what I said, but now, I'm not prepared to work in a place like that. I know what I'm prepared to tolerate and what I won't. I need to work somewhere where they can not only talk the talk, they can walk the walk.

Jesse felt completely differently. Her experiences, particularly the mobbing, had made her less likely to become involved with or supportive of others being bullied:

> I'm less likely to engage in political stuff. I was a person who stood up for others more than I will now. If I stick up for you, you'll leave me in the lurch, and I'm going to sink, and I can't be bothered with it. When I'm working, I'm invested in the place I'm working in. I feel a bit of exhaustion I may not have had if I hadn't dealt with all that.

8.6   Forgiveness

> It is the unjustness of things that I can't forgive. It's like an acceptance, and I don't want to accept that kind of injustice for anyone (Taylor).

During our conversations, I asked the champions about forgiveness. Did they think about it? Do they forgive the bullies, have tried, or think they should? Forgiveness is an interesting term. After reading many definitions, most suggest the person makes an intentional and voluntary decision to let go of negative emotions such as hatred or desire for revenge. Some definitions add that forgiving does not imply forgetting or condoning and is motivated by the person's desire for healing rather than appeasing the perpetrator. Some champions had not thought about forgiveness, and others had considered it quite a lot. Most found it very complex, generally with mixed feelings about whether they should forgive and what forgiving or otherwise meant for them and their bullying experiences.

Terry was not prepared to forgive and strongly believed the bullies did not deserve it:

I grew up being bullied at school, and it sits in me. No matter how successful I might be in my work, I will have a negative view of myself. Should I forgive people from back then that I'm in this situation? I don't think so. Should I forgive people doing it now and giving me a sense of not being good enough? No, I don't think so. I believe there are some horrendous arseholes out there who do not deserve my forgiveness. There are no excuses. If they wanted to reach out, it would take a lot of work. I don't think it's my job to clear the air. I wouldn't know what would happen if someone said, I'm sorry. I would accept an apology, but I don't think I would forgive. I see myself as hurt and as injured. I can understand someone who bullied me when they were 12 years old. We can have a conversation about that, and I can think of them as different people. In a workplace situation, meeting people who behave like this no way. They should know better. Common decency is common decency.

Over time, Andy thought less about the bully and its impact on her life. However, she still felt unable to forgive and would not likely do so without an apology or acknowledgement:

In one sense, I would like to, but no, I probably don't. I don't dwell on it. There are only a couple of people I would run over with my car, and she would be one of them. She's dropped down the list a little bit. I had a fucking good job, and she literally screwed me over. No doubt, these experiences have made me less forgiving. I don't think I need to forgive them for myself to move on from it. I don't know that my forgiving them will make it any better for me. For them to come and say sorry to me would be the one that would move me on more than anything. I hope there's some karma so you understand how you made me feel or anyone else that you did that too. I'm not perfect. Nobody is. But nobody needs to be made to feel like a piece of shit going to work. I was doing my job, and this is how you choose to behave. You should say sorry to me.

Shannon was able to forgive some bullies and not others, and when she could, she found forgiveness helpful in moving on:

I certainly feel very differently about the first incident. I've moved well and truly on. I have forgiven, and I've actually had that conversation. I needed to do that because I had trauma associated with that old workplace, which is terrible because I was there for 18 years. It was the only bad thing that ever happened. I left with a bitter taste and never got over it until I managed to have that conversation. I take this one personally. I've really been targeted by these two because they're more than aware that they're doing it.

Jesse made a fundamental distinction between personal and professional forgiveness:

I certainly forgive one bully. I can talk to her, and I'm okay about it. She had some real issues. With the other guy, I find it difficult to forgive. Still, I have reviewed his grants and articles and I am entirely professional. There is tension there. I sat behind him at a graduation ceremony, and he was just so tense, and I had a bit of a giggle. It's not really forgiven. I don't really care. He's quite successful, but I still see him as a little bit of an idiot, and I'm sure he knows that. I think, well, I don't really forgive you. You're a dick head. Do I dwell on it? No. Can I say hello to him in a crowd? Yes. Have I ever said anything about him, identifying him in any professional sphere? Never. So, I guess, in a professional sense, yes, I've forgiven him. In a personal sense, it was hurtful, ridiculous and unnecessary.

Rory and Sam would need to see something change in the bully, an apology or signs of remorse before they could forgive:

Rory: It depends on whether they're sorry for what they did. If someone came to me and said, "I'm so sorry, here is where I was wrong, this is what I should have done," that would be different. In the absence of that happening or even knowing what people are thinking, I think they're not sorry. I can forgive people who acknowledge what they did and feel sorry. There are people I haven't forgiven, and I can't imagine forgiving. I'm not in any way ready to forgive these people, and I'm not ready to completely move on. I'm ready to move forward, but I'm not ready to be over it. I'm not there yet.

Sam: That's an interesting question. I haven't thought about forgiveness. There's been a lot of sorrys that have come forth, but they have not been genuine. Forgiveness is an interesting word. I don't hate the person. I don't need her in my life as a friend or acquaintance. If things were to change and she acknowledged my existence in my position, that would be a win, win, win. I wouldn't care if there was an apology. It would allow me to get on with my job. It goes back to is this intentional? Is this personality? I look at forgiveness as somebody saying sorry, but there has to be a change of behaviour. And sorry doesn't always equate to that.

Alex felt that her capacity to forgive would show that she was the better person:

It's tough for me. I grew up in a Baptist environment. Even though I don't subscribe to a religious denomination, the concept of forgiveness is deeply rooted in the religion I was raised in. I can't say that I wouldn't forgive these people, even after what they did to me, because I like to believe that I'm a better person than they are. It's not a blank cheque. Many people think forgiveness is just a blank cheque, and if somebody says sorry, that wipes the slate. I still, to this day, have never received an apology from anyone there. If I ever got something meaningful and genuine, I would accept it because I never want to know what it is to be the type of human they are. The day I find myself unable to forgive a genuine decent apology is when I will be like them, and I never want that.

Lee described finding it more difficult to forgive and move on than she'd have expected, partly because of the apparent lack of consequences for the bully:

A little part of me tries to do that because the psychologist in me says, if you don't, it's you who suffers. The ongoing anger and resentment sit there and can be easily reactivated. Certainly, I forgive myself. I know I did everything according to policy, acted quickly, and did all the right things. I struggled more than I think I might have. I'm usually able to forgive a lot quicker. There's nothing on any level of her feeling any remorse or culpability, so it is hard, but at the same time, it's something I would like to get to. I'm surprised that it hasn't extinguished itself already. Talking to you about it, I don't have the heightened emotion or anger in my voice or body. But it hasn't completely been extinguished. If you'd asked me a year ago, I would have thought I would be over it by now. I'm really consciously, honestly aware that I haven't gotten to the point of full forgiveness yet. But I want to because I'm the one who will continue to feel it. She's probably having an espresso martini somewhere and not giving a shit. It's just stupid, but I'm not 100% there yet. I've done a lot of reflection and had some coaching. I've read practically everything in creation, and I know you can forgive but not forget. You can't just will it away, it's a process, and I'm doing it. I'd love to be passed it, to be frank.

Pat had similar thoughts about not forgetting and was consoled to some degree by a belief in karma:

I probably forgive, but I've got a memory like an elephant, and I'll never forget. Do I want to run her over now if I saw her walking in front of me? No. I firmly believe in karma, and I believe that somewhere down the line, she's going to pick the wrong person, and it's going to come around and bite her really hard on the backside.

The opportunity to make peace with one bully had helped Shannon in moving on:

It's funny because years down the track, I had the opportunity to work clinically with this manager, and we had quite a few conversations about clients. He never ever apologised to me. But he validated a lot for me. He said, "You know I really enjoy talking to you. You're a very skilled and wise clinician." I said, "Oh, thanks," and that was that. I was really grateful that he took the time to say that. I think that helped me move forward a bit.

Coming to some understanding of why bullies behaved as they did was necessary for some champions in the journey towards forgiveness:

Taylor: I've battled with the concept of forgiveness a lot. I try really hard to forgive people. I do that by trying to understand where they're coming from, and they're almost always coming from fear. So, trying to recognise and understand that they've been afraid helps me come to terms with their behaviour and what it has caused me. But as a person who was sexually assaulted as a child, I battle with forgiveness. That affects how you relate in almost every area of your life. So, it's too simplistic to think about it as just relating to bullying.

I can't forgive that, and it is the unjustness of things that I can't forgive. It's like acceptance, and I don't want to accept that kind of injustice for anyone. However, I can still value and love a person who has hurt me terribly. The hurt they have inflicted upon me hasn't undone the great work they have achieved. I can feel more kindly toward them and more forgiving if I focus on this. Can I ever really forgive them completely? I don't know, and I won't know until I draw my last breath. But, for the sake of myself, my family and my community, I think I can. I don't think constructive things can happen where poisonous thoughts and emotions exist, so I need to change my attitude towards the bullies and recognise their fear and pain. We need to appreciate them for their positive traits, abilities and what they have achieved.

Chris: This is a tricky one because if I think someone's behaviour stems from them having a particular personality structure, I don't excuse the behaviour. I'm not saying that the behaviour is acceptable. There's an element of they're wired in a particular way, and they're more likely to engage in specific behaviours. So you are more able to see why it occurs or how it has occurred. I may have to reflect on it more. I'm not trying to give those people a get-out-of-jail-free card because they should be accountable, and the system needs to hold them accountable. I'm more likely to forgive the person, the bully than I am to forgive the organisation if the organisation hasn't done the right thing.

Jordan: No, I don't forgive the bullies. I could forgive what they did to me personally if any of them had the decency to apologise or acknowledge the impact they had. What I absolutely can't and won't forgive is what their actions meant for the organisations involved, the profession and even more importantly, the people we are supposed to be caring for. No, I couldn't forgive that. However, they bother me a lot less now. One bully I used to see at conferences would smile sweetly and make small talk as though he had never stuck a dagger in my back, and I just couldn't cop it. Now I talk to him as I would any former colleague. I still think he is a nasty conniving man, but he doesn't bother me enough to ignore. I'm showing him I couldn't care less about him one way or the other. That's all I need to do. I don't need to forgive, and I won't.

For Rory, forgiveness was complicated by the indirect nature of her bullying experience, making it unclear who was responsible for what decisions or what their motivates might have been:

I don't know exactly who did and said what and what pressures were on them. So, I don't know who to blame and who is to be forgiven.

Taylor could forgive the bullying against her as an individual. However, she could not forgive what it had done to the broader professional community:

It's so unjust not to give all they and I had to give to our community. I find that unconscionable and unforgivable.

This resonates strongly with me. I can't forgive the roadblocks that bullies put in the way of good work purely because they don't like the person, or they want to get rid of them, or whatever their motives. I would much rather someone insult me to my face or direct any anger, jealousy, or whatever to me personally. At least it's on the table, and I know what the issue is. We are obliged to work together professionally and respectfully. The bullying that goes on in health services, universities and broader professional circles, I can never forgive.

I've thought about forgiveness a lot, and I still grapple with it, to be honest. I understand the definition and know it doesn't necessarily mean acceptance. Yet I still can't get out of my head that if I forgive people, I'm somehow saying what they did was okay or at least to shelve it somewhere. That's probably not logical, but I can't shift it in my thinking. I also understand that forgiveness is about doing things for yourself rather than others, and I get that. I'm sure that none of the bullies in my past would even give me a second thought. So, have I forgiven? Should I forgive? Can I forgive? I want to know the point of forgiving. Do I still think about the bullies and the bullying? Sometimes, more than I would like. Do I get still get angry? Again, sometimes. Do I need to forgive to move on? Having experienced bullying on several occasions by many people for over 20 years, I'm not sure what forgiving would do for me and the bigger picture. Have I moved on? I am no longer in a bullying environment, so from that perspective, yes, I have. Still, I haven't forgotten what was done to me, and I don't want to. What happened to me shaped me. It is now part of me. I have learned to live with it. What happened to the champions and what keeps happening to people in the health professions is wrong. People who are bullied because they're good at their job, because others feel threatened by them, or they don't want to be one of the girls or the boys, it is just so bloody wrong. No one should fear going to work and particularly not people who, in one way or another, contribute to the health and well-being of others. If forgiveness means I must set that aside, I will not forgive.

The Toxic Culture of Health

9

You can't tell us why you sacked her, but you're not addressing anything to us, and you've done nothing to change the culture (Lee).

Bullying is not just about individuals. Bullying on a large and continuous scale cannot occur unless the broader organisation allows the behaviours to continue. From the champions' stories, cultural problems are apparent. The broader system supports, condones and sometimes rewards bullying behaviours.

"The whole is more than the sum of its parts." This statement explains the dynamics of groups of people creating far more than the total of their individual contributions. It is a good starting point for understanding culture. An organisation's culture sets expectations about how people should behave with one another and the organisation as a whole. Expectations are communicated and supported by management and leadership teams. Employees come to understand what behaviours and actions are acceptable and what are not. Those who don't behave as expected are responded to according to those broader values. A positive workplace culture is crucial for people to be satisfied at work. It helps them feel safe and supported and able to use their skills and talents to reach their potential for themselves and, more importantly, the organisation.

The disjuncture between what is stated and what actually happens makes workplace culture difficult to understand and conform to. Preventing and dealing with workplace bullying requires policies with clear statements of zero tolerance and processes to follow where bullying occurs. If actions reflected policies, there would have been no book to write. Unfortunately, following processes and procedures have often led to more bullying. So, what does that say about the culture of healthcare organisations? This book would not be complete without considering the champions' perspectives on the workplace cultures of the organisations where the bullying occurred.

B. Happell, *Sickness in Health: Bullying in Nursing and other Health Professions*, https://doi.org/10.1007/978-3-031-49336-2_9

The champions clearly believed bullying was supported, or at least not acknowledged at an organisational level. Their experiences spoke to failure to act on bullying and a tendency to react defensively. They described a hierarchical culture dominated by competition, self-interest and a lack of leadership. The champions had at least initially been surprised that such a strong bullying culture would flourish in healthcare.

9.1   Problems with Leadership and Management

If you don't have a good culture and strong leaders who will pull these people aside and say, "That's not good enough here," it can happen anywhere in any workplace (Rory).

People who hold leadership positions are not necessarily leaders. Personal insecurity and an environment of competition can facilitate a bullying culture within an organisation. Instead of celebrating team successes, the so-called leader strives to keep people, particularly high achievers, under control. I recall a new head of school starting. From the moment she arrived, she appointed as many people she had previously worked with as possible. Some were close personal friends. Existing staff were treated as basically incompetent. She and her deputy set out to show staff how things should be done. Competitiveness played a big role. The deputy had big plans for her future there and wanted to position herself. Bringing others down was part of that. Perhaps she wanted to show the hierarchy that she had saved the school from its own incompetence. I don't have any problem with ambition. I do have a problem with backstabbing and humiliating and degrading people. I was only peripherally involved, but I saw and heard enough to realise that existing staff were bullied and stressed. A toxic culture of bullying had been established with surprising ease.

Rory and Sam discussed the importance of effective leadership for building a positive culture. Refusing to tolerate bullying is essential to stamping it out. Unfortunately, lack of training and preparation for leadership and management roles made the task so much harder:

Rory: If you don't have a good culture and strong leaders who will pull these people aside and say, "That's not good enough here," it can happen anywhere in any workplace. People don't have management training. They just get put into these positions.

Sam: When she first came here, I said if there is anything I have that she needs to let me know. We talked about research projects, and she talked about stuff she wanted to do and I said that's fantastic. We got along really, really well. And then she moved up the ladder. One of my theories is that she moved up too quickly. I think she's out of her depth. She's reactive and she's become a bit narcissistic in that, "this is what I've done, I've done this, I've done that." Whereas, you know, some of the nurses on the wards might have done something.

So-called leaders who did not lead fairly and equitably were all too common. Jesse saw a complex and problematic relationship between confidence and competence:

> The less competent you are. The more confident you are. If you're incompetent, you have no insight and think you're so competent. If you are competent, you understand that competence is on a continuum, and you will not always be the most competent. A stupid person thinks they know everything and can't go, "oh really. Is that true, okay? I might have to change my mind on that." They know everything.

Jordan talked about health professionals often being promoted based on their clinical skills and not being supported to develop and maintain skills for their new role:

> People get put into management positions for various reasons. Sometimes it's because they are good clinicians, which doesn't necessarily mean they're good managers. They get put in these positions and usually lack training or support. They don't know what they don't know. That's not an excuse to be a bully, but it does set that up more than if there was conscious attention to understanding what skills people need to be a manager.

Pat believed that employing younger staff who lacked experience and understanding contributed to problems with leadership and management:

> Don't give managerial positions to young people that don't have the common sense to run with those positions. You've got people in their late twenties that are given so much power to run programs or have positions where they're effectively playing with people's lives. In my case, I had this 30-something woman who wasn't married and didn't have kids. I don't think she understood what it would mean if I didn't have a job. I know that it's not her problem. Whereas someone with maturity and experience behind them sees things differently and approaches things differently.

9.2   Friendships and Being Liked

It was nothing about what I'd done. Someone there that didn't like me, and I knew that (Jesse).

In the chapter *How I responded,* champions talked about whether it was necessary to be liked in the workplace. I asked whether they felt there was a prevailing culture in health where those liked by management were treated differently from those not liked. Jesse talked about a strong culture of friendships being more important than experience and ability in deciding outcomes of job applications:

> It's absolutely who you know, not what you know. Some young people there were really good friends with the higher-ups and were given jobs well above their level. A job I applied for and didn't get. "He came up with this great model." It wasn't a great model. It was just what anyone would do. The rationale for promoting this person was empty, and I knew six thousand times as much. It was nothing about what I'd done. Someone there didn't like me, and I knew that. They told me I wasn't worth anything, which is an extraordinary thing to say to a person. They'd already decided this person was going to have the job.

Pat also observed that those who were liked were more likely to have opportunities to act in senior positions:

> At that hospital, it was about who was liked. So, any acting up into higher positions was whomever the powers that be liked.

Jordan described some of her previous workplaces as very social and friendship focused. Staying a bit distant from these interactions may have affected how her colleagues treated her:

> I don't go to work to make friends. In many environments I've worked in, particularly my last job, there was a real thing about being friendly. It was like one big social club. That's not my scene. I'm not one to pour over photos of grandchildren and bring in knitted booties or banana cakes. I'm not saying people shouldn't do it if they want to. It's not me; I won't force myself to have gratuitous friendships. I've always been polite and pleasant, attended farewells and indulged in some small talk. It's just not what I go to work for. I'd rather get my work done. When I make friends at work, it's genuine. It's because I like them, not because it's in my interest to hang out with them because they're my boss or might give me a job one day. That has cost me in some circles, not sitting down for endless morning teas and talking about baking or children. People have trouble separating friendship from professionalism and collegiality.

Alex talked about the culture of friendship as determining who was accepted as part of the group and who was bullied because they weren't:

> They are a very incestuous group and want everyone to be a certain way. There's a big drinking culture, a culture of them all going out together, and I wasn't part of that. I didn't allow anybody access to my private life, which was a problem for them. You're either with them or against them, including bullying behaviour. You have to partake in that, and you have to decide early on to be a torturer or be tortured. That's not my personality. I can't be mean to somebody for no reason. People I thought were nice, you watched them very quickly become horrible. My solicitor has ten clients from the service. It's a hotbed for work cover cases because of the culture.

9.3   Competition, Self-interest and Insiders

> Health jobs these days, a lot are contract positions, so it's about saving your own butt, so you've got a job. So, people tend to push others under the bus (Pat).

I find the academic environment in my discipline very toxic. There is so much competition, and it depends a lot on who likes whom rather than what people can achieve or contribute. This spills over from the universities into professional organisations. When selecting keynote speakers for conferences, it's more about who the influential people get along with than who has made the most significant contribution to the area. I've seen a strong competitive edge even when you work for the same place. When I started a new job, a colleague, at the same level as me, said quite openly she had not wanted me at that university because "it's a very small paddock." We had known each other for many years and worked on projects together, and I believed we had mutual respect. At least she was honest. I found it very sad. What must it be like to want to promote your own success at the expense of the organisation and profession more broadly? She had a management role, so she could have relished having someone with a solid track record working for the same place. I've seen people selected for roles with virtually no transparency about the process. Two senior positions on an editorial board went to former colleagues of the editor. Were they the best people for the job? Who would know? There was no information about how many people applied and what criteria were used to select. The Committee was simply asked to ratify the appointments. I expressed concern about the credentials of one applicant, and my concerns were dismissed. Competitiveness and nepotism are just so destructive for our profession. We have some very talented people, including the bullies. If we worked together, we could do so much more. That's the part that frustrates me the most. "Jobs for the girls," I call it. Such a shame to see a female-dominated profession taking on some of the worst aspects of masculine culture.

Sam and Andy saw a highly competitive environment with staff who wanted to climb the ladder:

Sam: I am supposed to gather data to present to improve some things in my area. I know he'll present them as his, not mine, and that's fine because I'm not about the accolades. I'm just about getting the job done. I don't want to climb up the ladder. I want to deliver the best care, which works to my detriment in many ways. It means that people at the top aren't really aware of the work I do. They see me as what the senior nurse portrays me as.

Andy: There is a big culture of climbing over someone to get somewhere. Even within our department, on the surface, it all looks great, but as you get to know people, you discover that the same thing goes on. People are treated differently depending on who you are and who you know.

Pat believed the competitive and insecure environment of the healthcare workforce was a possible motive:

Health jobs these days, a lot are contract positions, so it's about saving your own butt, so you've got a job. So, people tend to push others under the bus so they're not victimised by the bully.

9.4 Hierarchies

Health care is a brutal industry because of the hierarchical organisation of these institutions and the disempowering bureaucracy and professional conditions (Terry).

The strong hierarchical nature of health care was considered a significant contributor to the bullying culture. Terry talked about the organisational complexity that makes health workplaces particularly susceptible to bullying:

Health care is a brutal industry because of its historical heritage, the hierarchical organisation of these institutions and the disempowering bureaucracy and professional conditions. It's got hierarchical decision-making. It's got professional groups that are continually fighting for privilege and power. A lot of the conflicts between people, up and down in the hierarchies, are very complex already, even before you start bullying each other. It's as if you've already started a fight simply because you belong to one mob compared to another. There are some levels of entitlement to be able to bully someone in this system that you don't see elsewhere because it's less complicated. You bring so much with you into a conversation that you wouldn't be doing if you were an engineer or a software developer. I don't just go to work and fix the thing. It's important to me to accomplish what I'm accomplishing. People who bring a lot of who they are as people into their work functions run a risk of getting hurt if they end up in bad situations. Whereas if you treat your job as a place to make money, there would be less risk.

Rory also described a very hierarchical structure made even worse by the fierce competition in medical training programs, complicated reporting relationships and busy, stressful environments:

It's very hierarchical. Even just looking at a ward round. You've got your consultant and registrars and all the way down to your medical students. There are limited places on training programs, and because the people who are doing your assessments and providing you with references to get on to training programs are also the people who sign your overtime, it gets very muddy. On top of that, you've got busy, stressful work environments where you're dealing with people's health and sick patients and, often, difficult conversations, and the correct treatment isn't always obvious. You've got different departments. You're making referrals to people who are busy, stressed and have other priorities. Then you throw nurses, allied health, and everyone else into the mix, who also have various roles, experience and power. It can get very messy very quickly.

Taylor made an interesting observation about the impact of hierarchies on the culture of organisations she had worked for. In her peer role, she found herself frequently called upon for support by nurses and medical staff, many of whom had been bullied by their colleagues:

I kept track over one week of how much time I spent supporting nurses. My role was manager of peer work. I added how much time I spent supporting nurses, doctors and other health staff who were bullied, intimidated and struggling with mental health issues. They never talked to me about mental health issues in relation to the patients. It was always about their peers, other staff members, nurses, registrars and doctors. Registrars would also talk to me about being bullied by nurse unit managers and doctors. About 27% of my time in one week went into supporting clinical staff. I think that they came to me because there is a real strength in shared vulnerability. It gives them permission and a feeling of safety to share their vulnerability with me.

The perceived higher status of medical practitioners sometimes created a sense of entitlement to be a bully:

Andy: Our doctors think they are God because they are cardiologists. When you have guys coming to their fellowship, they always say, "If I turn into an arsehole like him, please tell me." And as they finish their fellowship, they are exactly like that. And we say to them, "You're turning. Look at how you are speaking. Listen to your behaviour." But by that point, they don't care and are just arseholes to us.

Jesse: I had a colleague who had this lovely partner. He was doing psychology because he wanted to get into medicine. Then he did medicine, and he became the snootiest bastard and actually wouldn't talk to me anymore because I wasn't a doctor. It just really turned him. I've taught a lot of doctors. I think they're indoctrinated to think they're pretty special. Because I've worked in population health, I was always made to feel a little bit lesser because I wasn't a doctor, but I didn't take that personally. I'm, like, yeah, whatever.

9.5   Not Dealing with Bullies

> There was a lot of anxiety and meetings about workplace culture and bullying, and nothing changed. It's always going to be the same (Andy).

The champions told of many instances where bullying was tolerated and even rewarded, resulting in toxic cultures. Lee described working with a bully who created considerable distress for many staff. Despite this being known to management, she remained in the organisation, sometimes moved sidewise, without operational responsibilities and ultimately came back into managerial roles to repeat the behaviours time and time again:

> She really harassed different people, they never really got rid of her, but in some context, they put her back in her cage. Then the leadership structures were changed, and within five or six years, she'd come back out again and be quite toxic. They constantly didn't address it, and by that stage, she got rid of nearly everyone I knew who was really good.

Chris and Pat had similar experiences of the bully being supported by the organisation and, therefore able to continue the behaviour unchecked:

Chris: Unfortunately, the person had the backing of the organisation and didn't tell the truth about lots of things that went on. They've been doing this for many years and getting away with it. I later found out the original workplace did get rid of her, but not before she had, on paper, 18 other people complained of bullying from her. So, this is long-standing behaviour that she's engaged in. She's still there. She got away with it. She has continued to move into positions higher up the ladder. So, you're unlikely to change your behaviour if you get rewarded for it.

Pat: The CEO certainly supported the bully boss. She was promoted. People have made complaints, and what do you do? You promote her. Pat her on the head. From what I understand, she worked for another hospital and did exactly the same thing. I said, "Did nobody check her references?" "Did they give her glowing references to get rid of her?" They feel that she was headhunted to get rid of certain staff on our team.

Lee also believed bullies were often valuable to the organisation for getting rid of people that were no longer wanted.

> The leadership and the management want these people there. They're their Rottweilers. "You enact this plan to get rid of the deadwood here."

Chris and Rory believed bullies were more likely to be backed by the organisation if they were successful in their jobs:

Chris: This person's very powerful. They can be very charming and had achieved a lot for the organisation. I do believe if the person wasn't achieving things and empire-building successfully, then they probably wouldn't have backed this person the same way. There were a lot of successes that occurred because of her, new opportunities and doors opening. So, they probably thought, we're prepared to put up with some bad behaviour because look at all this good stuff over here. No one ever said it, but I do think they had awareness because somebody else before me had the same experience from this person. She had also gone to management, and they had basically said, "yep, we're never talking about this again".

Rory: I had a consultant who undermined me in front of a patient the other day, it's not the first time, and I've seen her doing it to others. I spoke to the director about it because I'd rather they know this is a problem early. My description of events was certainly accepted as the truth, but I felt disappointed by the response. I was told she's a good consultant. That's one of those problems in healthcare. They don't say, "let me look into it and see whether anything is going on or whether they need a bit of performance management." Yeah, but they're a good consultant." I actually said something back." This is someone who has real issues communicating with other doctors and nurses. And does that really make her a good consultant?

Andy talked about a very defensive response from the organisation when concerns about bullying were raised in the staff survey. Rather than welcoming the information and dealing with the issues presented, a bad situation became worse:

> The organisation had a staff survey. It was supposed to be anonymous, but we were one small group by itself on the survey results. So, they knew it came from us. We were harassed by the senior managers. They bullied us into having meetings about what we wrote in the survey. We had to tell them why. We're saying we're getting bullied from above, and you want us to meet with the people who are bullying us? We're not going to do that. We were directed to attend meetings, and if we didn't, disciplinary action would be taken against us. These meetings were to be facilitated by the people that were deemed to be the bullies. It tells us to shut up, basically. No one was really listening, so we will never ever fill in that document ever again.

Lee was trying to let the new boss know how the toxic culture remained even though the bully was gone and no action had been taken to address it. The response from the new boss was startling:

Things were so terrible, things that happened to me, and no one came down and said, "are you okay?" No one did anything. So, I said to her, "I don't feel that I am valued by you. There are things that went on. There's lots of things that happened, none of which have ever been addressed. I know that I gave you millions of papers and good examples from this place and that place where they've done it well. I gave you papers from the university, and then we never met again. I find it very hard to commit to a place that has not supported me." She was shocked. A couple of times, I said how hard I found things from last July. I'd go to tell her something horrible, she'd cry, and I'd be consoling her and it would be really fucking annoying. This is not very helpful, but now I have to manage other people with emotions.

Apathy from organisations was identified by champions as a significant barrier. Their failure to act often facilitated the behaviour continuing. For Sam, this made it more difficult to have faith in her senior manager:

I believe certain aspects of what the senior manager was saying were genuine. But, in the same breath, I don't trust that level of management because these issues have been taken to her many times by many people, the way that the senior nurse treats people. Nothing has ever really been done about it that I am aware of. The senior manager suggested I write a letter and put bullying on the table, and then she has to address it. But we all know that wouldn't go anywhere.

No action was taken when Andy raised concerns about the response to the survey results. Nothing had changed, and she didn't believe it would in the future:

I got the union in, and they tried to assist us because of this intimidatory process. We had debriefing meetings. We put our points of view across, how our doctors talk to us, how they treat us and how things are run by the department head and nurse unit manager. But nothing ever changed. Nothing's changed ever since then. So, there was a lot of anxiety and meetings about workplace culture and bullying, and nothing changed. It's always going to be the same.

When Shannon made complaints about bullying, not only was no action taken, but she also exposed a lack of information exchange within management itself, which no doubt gave fuel to the bullying culture:

They won't performance manage. It's been going on for three years. This is the third lot of senior clinicians they've gone through because of these two. I can see, organisationally, where the buck stops. And it does never flow up to the general manager. She's not informed. And so, she's gap-filling.

When another staff member left and supported Shannon's reports of bullying, a decision was made to change the organisational structure and make the two staff concerned redundant. The lack of communication was to continue with Shannon and her colleague being asked to be complicit:

When the redundancy talk occurred, my colleague and I were asked to keep it confidential because my manager wasn't informed. They put us in a really difficult situation. Unfortunately, she doesn't know about the changes coming. They've kept her out of the loop. I think it's cruel because we know. I think they're excusing themselves by saying we're protecting her from the stress of it. It just means that somewhere down in the wash, it will come out that we already know about this. And that we've kept it from her, and that's not transparent practice.

Similarly, when Sam's manager did propose some action, her suggestions were more about manipulating the situation rather than dealing with it head-on:

I met with the general manager, and she asked me how things were going, and I said, "they're not." The bully went to a secondment. So, the general manager asked me to set up meetings with the person acting, get my name on all the distribution lists, get myself invited to key meetings, send this email and bcc her into it. I said, "that feels underhanded, and I don't work that way". She said, "Well, I think we have to do it this way." I met with the person acting. He put me on all those lists. The general manager told me I had to get him to diarise monthly meetings with the bully, and she cancelled them. She directed the bully to meet with me, but she would cancel the meetings. I hadn't had a meeting with her for seven months.

Terry, after witnessing and experiencing so much bullying, felt helpless about the behaviours being continually ignored:

I've had conversations with some colleagues about how to stop the bullying culture that seems to be allowed, and I don't know how to. It's ignored by the senior management. It's flat-out ignored. The university and the hospital are organisations of ignorance. They ignore these problems.

I can relate to so many of these experiences. The culture of health is jam-packed with bullying. It's so much a part of these organisations many probably don't recognise it as bullying. It's probably seen as normal practice, although when they're out to get somebody, and the tactics are extreme, I find it hard to believe they wouldn't know what they're doing. It's so endemic that bullies have often been bullied themselves. Due to a complete and total lack of awareness that baffles me with health professionals, particularly mental health professionals, they transfer that down the line to someone else. That happened to me. I had an excellent relationship for quite some time with the senior nurse until a change in her management line, and the relationship turned sour. She could deal with things and be pleasant and collegial when all was well. Once that changed, she didn't cope, and perhaps she was looking for someone to blame and I conveniently filled that space. That is no excuse. One thing I've learnt from the bad managers I've had over the years is never to transfer your crap to people who work with or for you. I've always been very aware of that. I genuinely believe I continued to treat my team members and colleagues with respect, despite whatever was going on for me.

From my experience, there is no willingness to communicate openly and effectively and talk about concerns as they arise. Why don't we have conversations about how things are going? If I'm doing something wrong or the rules have changed, let's talk about it. In my experience, that rarely happened. It was all about surreptitiously backstabbing. Why do the communication skills all health professionals possess go out the window when it comes to dealing with colleagues? It doesn't make any sense to me. Unfortunately, this lack of communication fuels a culture of bullying and toxicity.

When action was taken, and the bully in Lee's workplace was removed, an immediate solution to bullying was found. However, the underlying culture of the organisation that allowed the behaviour to continue was not addressed:

> "You can't tell us why you sacked her, but you're not addressing anything to us, and you've done nothing to change the culture." Some of those people who were enabled and empowered by her are still sitting there, not full-on bullies, not in power, but they're splitting, they're difficult, they're mobbing, they're doing their own little thing, and for an organisation that's literally got mentally healthy workplace programs that we teach to people. I want them to come into line and behave. I want them to apologise to us. I want them to offer us things. These people who took time off because they were being bullied by her, I want them to have their sick days reinstated. The Board should know better. What would we tell another organisation to do, given we promote mentally healthy workplaces? It's not just ironic. It's hurtful.

Alex talked about the life-threatening impact of failing to address the organisational culture that supported bullying:

> They haven't ever had a Royal Commission for the Ambulance Service. They desperately need one. I think they've been a part of 12 enquiries now. When I testified, I didn't know about the lady who hanged herself after being bullied so savagely in the service. I've read the horrific letter she wrote to them pleading before she took her life. I've read some horrific things, and I understand I will never change these people. This has been going on much longer than I realised. The last thing I said to them was that if they didn't do something and allowed the Ambulance to continue to self-police and self-regulate, somebody else would die. They average one employee a quarter now taking their own lives. It wasn't long after that another man hanged himself in his paramedic uniform to make a statement. It's a culture that is ingrained there.

When Taylor became a whistle-blower, revealing the serious criminal behaviour of a staff member, there was no support for her within the organisation:

> When I told my boss what I was going to do, they said: "All hell is going to break loose here. I have to try and keep this service running. I won't be able to support you in public." They meant in front of the other staff. They said, "I will support you in here behind closed doors, but I won't be able to support you out there because I've got to keep this service running." So, I told my staff they must keep themselves safe and not come near me. "Don't be seen even speaking to me." I would have to manage it by myself and protect the person that had made the allegation.

Lee noted how difficult it can be for organisations to deal with bullies, who are often very skilled at controlling the environment:

> Workplace psychopaths with their really toxic culture in place, you have to be careful. They're good at it, they've gone to lawyers three or four times over, they're skilled. You have to be incredibly careful.

In a new role, Jordan was trying to manage staff who totally undermined her with no apparent consequences:

> I'd started this new role as a director of a research centre. Before accepting the position, I'm told I have a full-time project officer and a half-time clinician-researcher. Virtually as the project officer introduced herself, she told me that she's really busy for the next six months writing report for a project, she got a few thousand dollars in funding for, and won't be able to do anything else much. Okay great. The clinician-researcher says much the same. He's very busy in the other half of his role and won't be able to do much else. Apart from an assistant, they were the only staff I had. I talked about it with my boss, and she said, "don't worry, the project office is retiring in six months, and you can get somebody else in her place, leave her go. Not much good rocking the boat." She said the clinical researcher should spend 50% of his time doing research under my direction. I tried to talk to him about this, and he became very defensive and antagonistic. I wasn't asking him to do my research work. I was offering to help him to determine what he wanted to do for his future career and write up publications from his PhD. He wasn't having a bar of it. I even organised a three-way meeting where the boss said he needed to spend 50% of his time with the centre. Nothing changed. When I asked him to do a session for a workshop, he later cancelled because he had something else on that day for his other job. That was the last straw. I had had enough of the blatant disrespect he had gotten away with for nearly 18 months. I told my boss, "I don't care if his position isn't replaced; I don't want him here anymore". So, he was moved on. I couldn't get over the audacity. It totally undermined my position, and that is bullying. It is definitely toxic, and the culture supported that.

Bullies become powerful because they can. I have been gobsmacked at how bullies intimidate people at all levels of the organisation and get away with it. One colleague stands out. Grandstanding and blatant abuse of power was his pattern of behaviour with colleagues. It was extraordinary to see how intimidated staff were, even people I considered strong and assertive. I was a member of the school ethics committee. He took exception because some committee members had let their students know the outcomes straight after the meeting. He stated this was inappropriate because it gave some students an unfair advantage. At the next meeting, we were told we could not tell students until they were informed officially. This was taken for granted until I pointed out that every staff member has the right to attend the meetings at any time, so there was no issue with informing students. I had to really push to get them to change their minds. He then complained about how feedback was reported, and we were all expected to sign our names to our own comments. Again, accepted without consideration. I objected strongly because we make decisions as a committee, not as individuals. Undoubtedly, he would have targeted people who made comments he didn't like. He had history, and this was going to be allowed! So as much as I found him an overbearing and unacceptable bully, I was more concerned about the response of others, including those in charge of the organisation.

In Terry's experience, organisational bullying involved setting targets that couldn't be achieved. These expectations were preventing him from engaging in the quality and type of research he was interested in:

> I see the bullying and what people are supposed to deal with. It's getting worse. It's humiliating to be asked to accelerate beyond what's possible. The structural demands at the university are impossible. They're not healthy for someone like me. I'm supposed to generate

X amount of dollars every year. I'm supposed to write X amounts of successful applications for competitive funding. At the same time, I'm expected to have a huge research output. I'm supposed to be a teacher and of service to the university, and I'm supposed to have a job at a hospital. I can't do it all and haven't met anyone who does. I feel I'm caught up in a hamster wheel where I'm running faster and faster, and I'm expected to re-invent myself again and again, and I can't see where it would stop. I'm also in a temporary position. When I'm being evaluated, it may be an issue. When I look at my CV, this whole set-up has pushed my research in a direction where I'm not thinking brilliant new thoughts. I'm just doing almost insignificant research because that's what the university wants. They want quantity over quality. I don't have the opportunity to do the fine and deep thinking I associate with a professor at a university. This is slowly draining me. I'm on the road to burnout.

9.6   Surprised at Bully Culture

Within my profession, there are some of the highest rates of bullying. Many nurses will be on the receiving end of bullying. Why, why can't we look after each other (Chris)?

Several champions expressed surprise at the bullying culture in health, particularly given the supposed caring nature of health professions, as Chris described:

Yes, absolutely. And it's still something that I find really upsetting. On the one hand, I'm really proud that I'm a nurse. I think it's a great profession. There is lots I love about it. But I'm really embarrassed to say that within my profession, there are some of the highest rates of bullying. Many nurses will be on the receiving end of bullying. Why, why can't we look after each other? Because I'm not wired like that at all. Throughout this most recent bullying, I constantly rang people and checked in with them. How are you going? What's your self-care? If you're not coping, remember you've got the employee assistance program and remember you can go to your GP. Make sure you do something nice tonight. The reality is the more you read into it and read research papers, there are particular personality structures. In the most recent one, you could see that she thoroughly enjoyed hurting people. You could see the dopamine hit literally taking place. And so, people with those types of personality structures can sometimes be drawn into these areas of work.

Andy was particularly surprised this hadn't changed with the new generation of nurses who had not had the same rigid, hierarchical approach to their education:

People go into caring professions because they want to help people, they want to care, and support. As the generations have come through, I find it even more bizarre. They weren't treated terribly in the wards and in nursing education like us hospital-trained people. The new millennia have a voice, but it's still out there. I don't understand. Older generations like myself were trained not to say anything, do what the doctor said, and not respond.

Although bullying clearly occurred in other professions and occupations, Pat still found it at odds with health professionals who are supposed to be caring and should have the skills to reflect on and consider their own behaviour:

It is surprising. When I was working at the children's hospital in the social work department, I thought, "You're social workers, and you're bullying other social workers." Why go into the profession if that's the type of personality that you have? I can't explain it. It is surprising.

I couldn't agree more. Even after all the times I've been bullied and seen and heard about bullying from my colleagues, I still wonder how this can be. What surprises me is that health professionals, surely most of them anyway, come into this field because they want to make a positive difference in people's lives. They want to improve people's health and well-being. So why, then, do they become bullies? How do they not see the impact of their behaviour on other humans? I find that still, to this day, the big question that I haven't been able to answer. In my speciality area of mental health, it is particularly perplexing. These professionals are responsible for ensuring positive outcomes for extremely vulnerable people. Academics who teach empathy but display absolutely none of that to their colleagues defy logic to me. The bully from the ethics committee taught conflict resolution. We used to laugh about that, although it really wasn't funny. I find myself looking at these bullies and thinking what is wrong with you that you can't have a decent conversation? That you can't deal with differences of opinion? That you can't tell people what you're concerned about instead of carrying on with passive-aggressive tactics? As much as it hurts, it fascinates me.

Rory had seen enough of it that the shock had worn off. However, she was still surprised and disappointed by the lack of humanity from many health professionals:

> I'd been in the hospital long enough by then to see all the power dynamics, and I was surprised by just how unprofessional it felt and the absolute lack of transparency. I was surprised by how inhumane it felt and how they treated another professional, but I wasn't entirely shocked. By that stage, I had many other people's awful stories in various rotations and hospitals over the years. I think I was surprised and disappointed at how different it can be. It's like a work face for the patients and then something different when you're treating your colleagues.

9.7   Strategies

> The day he decides to look at the people in that organisation and say, "we don't do this anymore. We don't behave this way anymore …" The first person that loses their job … it'll stop (Alex).

We all know that bullying is a problem, but we know much less about what to do about it. In our last conversation, I asked the champions what ideas or strategies might help in changing the culture that facilitates bullying. Terry did not believe bullying could be fixed and could only be moderated with effective leadership:

> I don't think it can be fixed. I think it's part of the way humans get organised. We can mitigate it to some extent, and I would see it as a leadership issue. The type of organisation is envisioned and put into place by the absolute top of the system and then passed down to the rest. Bullying is part of the toxicity of the hierarchical, violent mental health care organisations we have had for centuries. We work in a dehumanising environment where people's context and lives are ripped away from them, allowing us to deal with each other as professionals in some of the same ways.

On the other hand, Alex believed culture change was possible and well within grasp. She suggested thinking otherwise was purely a cop-out:

> One of the biggest things I've seen, especially in government organisations, that is so annoying is talking about how hard it is to change the culture. It's really not. The day he decides to look at the people in that organisation and say, "we don't do this anymore. We don't behave this way anymore, and we have zero tolerance for it". The first person that loses their job, it'll stop. That has to start at the top because people at the bottom are powerless. I tried to change things, and look what happened to me. I can't do it. It's got to be someone with power and influence. I don't think they want to change it because it gives them elements to control people. That's how they've always worked. That's how they manoeuvre through their careers, having this ability to torment people.

Although their responses are opposing, I agree with both Terry and Alex to some degree. My son was bullied at primary school. At the start of the next school year, I discussed this with his new teacher. "Not in my class," she said, and she was right. Not once was he bullied that year. The next year with a new teacher, it started again. At the same time, I understand the complexities Terry has described. Large organisations have such complicated management structures, and then there's the issue of whether they want to change and are prepared to do what it takes to make bullying a thing of the past.

Addressing Bullying

> It can be addressed by showing a great deal of compassion and intention to get good outcomes. Not sweeping it under the carpet. Listening … and respecting what is being said (Taylor).

Taylor believed that bullying needed to be addressed at the time in a positive and supportive way that could be a growth opportunity for all concerned. This view had been reinforced at her current workplace:

> We will, perhaps forever, because people are people, and experience relationships where there can be intimidation or bullying. So long as that is addressed, it can be a learning experience for everyone and be very healing and build further resilience. If managed well, it can be used as an opportunity for growth, reflection, understanding, trust and improved relationships. That's been my experience at my current job. It can be addressed by showing a great deal of compassion and intention to get good outcomes. Not sweeping it under the carpet. Listening, deeply listening and respecting what is being said. Recognising that the different people involved will have different background experiences and different conceptions of what has happened. Help all involved to feel safe enough to open their minds to engage with and see how the other person was feeling, what triggered it and try and find understanding of the person initiating the bullying or intimidation, where they may have been coming from. So, there could be an aim of healing traumas and relationships.

Sam and Chris also talked about the need to bring bullying out into the open:

Sam: The only way to fix it is to bring it out, and I think that's starting to happen
          now. Making people aware is one way, and making a safer process to call
          it out. If we could make it easier but not so easy. When you report it, you
          have to go up so high, and the fact you're going up that high is intimidating
          and nobody wants to listen unless someone has punched you or raped you.
          People high up don't want to acknowledge it because it's their house.
Chris: We still have such a long way to go in our society in terms of having the
          right procedures and processes in place for when it happens. They need the
          training; they need support mechanisms in place that say this is what we
          do. It's still a little bit of that age-old attitude that it is easier to say to the
          victim, "I'm sure it's not as bad as all that," instead of having the conversa-
          tion and saying I'm so sorry you're having that experience, I'd like to
          understand more and know how I can help. People are just not equipped to
          have those conversations. I think so many things have to be addressed in
          our society to make inroads. Having these conversations with you could
          mean that people read your book and can have a better understanding of
          things and be protection for someone. Who knows?

Andy believed good communication would be a key component in addressing
bullying, providing staff with the opportunity to be heard and supported:

> The thing that really makes a big difference is communication. Everyone's clear, everyone's
> able to speak freely and confident to say, "I don't like what you're saying, and I'm going to
> speak to the boss about it," or just go and speak to the boss, but feel you're being heard, and
> something can change. Feeling supported. I know people have gone to my boss, and it's just
> like, suck it up. He's not skilled. He doesn't want to do anything about it, so frustration
> builds and it creates more of an uncomfortable situation.

Taylor suggested the need to openly talk about emotions in the workplace to
facilitate effective communication and break down the silence around bullying:

> We should be talking about emotions a lot more in workplaces and be accepting of emotions
> as not being unprofessional. Words like love, graciousness, care, compassion, fondness and
> concern should be used and respected in the workplace. They should be traits that are wel-
> comed, engaged with, accepted and sought after.

Several champions referred to the need for management and leadership training
to identify and respond to bullying and its impact. For example, Lee saw bullying as
needing a management response equivalent to that of a physical disaster:

> At the corporate level, there needs to be training and education to offer people some sup-
> port. If it had been a workplace physical accident like a chemical spill, they would have
> come in and done something. We had the psychological equivalent, and because they didn't
> want to apologise, because it looks like we were liable, we don't want to do anything. It is
> reprehensible.

Pat saw the need for better processes for receiving an accurate and honest account of performance before employing managers, something that could minimise the likelihood of bullying:

> One of the biggest problems is when people are applying for jobs, they give their references, and when people check references and their boss lies. "They're fantastic managers, great managers." They're not because this bitch, what she did to the team, she had done to the team at her last job. If they'd done their job properly and the last place had been honest, the train wreck could have been avoided.

Accepting that recruitment strategies are far from foolproof when it comes to detecting bullies, Lee saw the need for processes to remove the bully and protect the targets:

> You are better off having good processors to kick them out. The mechanisms to protect people once they become unmasked and move them on or help them to redeem themselves. Do your best not to hire them but knowing that that's hard, make sure the processes are there to get rid of them straight away and then support and do damage control afterwards.

Rory suggested the need for consequences for bullying and a process to avoid bullies moving from one organisation to another without their behaviour being identified:

> There needs to be more consequences. We need to start firing people who are bullies. There are just no consequences, as far as I can see. Once you've had a bullying complaint that's been proven, not to say that you can't have a job elsewhere and you can't reform, but I think that that needs to be on your record so that other hospitals know they need to keep a really close eye on you.

Processes for Reporting

> There needs to be something set up where you report bullying that isn't directly to the person that affects your training and job prospects (Rory).

Andy described a system for reporting bullying anonymously. Someone from HR would chat with the person informally over a cup of coffee. While it had produced some positive benefits, Andy had seen it used when not warranted, completely devastating the person involved:

> The hospital has implemented an assistant called We care, where you can anonymously make a complaint about someone, and it has to be addressed. We've had doctors who were complete assholes, and the We Care system has had them pull their socks up and not speak so nastily, and then they get back to their habits. It has good benefits, and it can be devastating. It's a no-blame thing. That's what they say. There's no consequence in your record, but for the person, there still is. It's happened to a friend, and he's completely devastated. It got him to the point of near suicide. I firmly believe he didn't do anything worth complaining

about to this level. He's had someone speak to him, and he's worried, "you're going to think that I'm some person who says and does the wrong thing, and you have this picture of me now." All he did was tell a colleague that something she was saying was incorrect and go to the policy and look it up. He's pretty fragile, and it still affects him. You have no right of reply because it's all anonymous except, of course, within a small department. We know that this girl has done it on several occasions.

Rory saw the need for an independent process to cut through the complex power differentials so doctors aren't discussing bullying with people they are dependent on for career progression:

There needs to be a separation between who's writing your assessments and your references and who you go to discuss issues such as being bullied. People often don't address it because they're trying to get into a training program or need a good reference. There needs to be something set up where you report bullying that isn't directly to the person that affects your training and job prospects.

9.8   Making ilt Happen

Whether it's Parliament, a hospital, or a university, the mindset has to shift. "Yes, we have bullying, and this is what we are doing, and we are proud of what we are doing" (Jordan).

Alex, Chris, Jordan and Rory gave their ideas for turning strategies into action to create awareness of and address bullying at the broader level:

Alex: It needs to be a national initiative. We need to de-stigmatise mental health. I've worked in health, and I didn't have the information about mental health that I have now. I learnt what I know by being a mental health patient. Education has got to be there.

Chris: So much of it comes down to detecting it early. We have programs and schools teaching young people what bullying looks like and its impact on relationships. You hope that doing those things younger and younger will have a positive impact on the emotional development of some of our young people. You also hear of programs being utilised to teach the younger aged about empathy. If people can empathise with another person, will that deter them from wanting to harm that person? You hope.

Jordan: This needs to come from the very top. With all that's going on in Parliament, this is the best opportunity we've had to do something, really do something. The conversation has started, so it's time to say, "Okay, we're going to fix this." Let's listen to the experts. What causes bullying? What stops it? How do we change the culture? There definitely needs to be an independent reporting system. People who've been bullied are shattered and exhausted and need somewhere to go. Someone that will listen and take them seriously. We need to recognise subtle bullying, exclusion, ignoring, blocking and all of that. The bullying needs to be investigated independently, with the aim of resolution. There is such a culture of sweeping bullying under the table. That must stop. Whether it's Parliament, a hospital, or a university, the mindset has to shift. "Yes, we have bullying, and this is what we are doing, and we are proud of what we are doing."

Rory: A few hospitals need to take the lead, and maybe others will follow suit. The regional places that may be struggling to recruit doctors will always be problematic because they're not going to want to address it. Ultimately, you'd think it would be in their best interest, even if they struggle in the short term, because it'll be easier to retain staff.

Chris previously held a casual role teaching nursing students about bullying. She hoped this could make them more aware. This had provided her with a way to make sense of her own experiences:

> I've lectured at uni into the undergraduate nursing degree. We would talk about bullying and the nursing profession and get students to read the literature and latest research about workplace bullying. I think we're trying to do much more now about understanding that within the nursing profession, particularly, there are really high rates of bullying, harassment and other forms of behaviours. We're trying to get better at educating people about what it looks like so that you don't experience it for two years before you go, hang on, "I'm experiencing workplace bullying." Then, hopefully, people can get clued in faster and are clearer about their options for trying to do something about it.

Before asking that question of the champions, I had written my thoughts about strategies. After listening to their ideas, I have added many more, my thoughts enriched by theirs. So, the culture of health? Something must give. There needs to be a complete review of how health organisations deal with bullying, particularly the subtle kinds that can be much harder to demonstrate. As the champions have suggested, there needs to be an independent process where any complaint someone makes or concern they raise is dealt with. Not in how HR deals with it, by sweeping it under the carpet or turning it around on the person who raised the issue. It doesn't necessarily have to be punitive, at least not at the beginning. It can be more like Taylor's experience, where someone sits with the target and the person they believe has bullied or harassed them, and the behaviours are discussed. It doesn't have to be about blame. It could be okay, "this is how Deirdre feels about some of the ways you are managing her." The boss considers and listens, hopefully with the support and encouragement of the independent person. It can be a beginning process to work these things through. It would need to be something that couldn't just be ignored. The alleged bully would need to report back on how practices had changed, and feedback would need to come from the target regarding how things were working. It wouldn't be foolproof, of course. Still, it would be a bloody good start and a hell of a lot better than what we have now, which is nothing other than a biased and reactionary HR system and a largely toothless industrial system. The system is broken, and it needs to be fixed. These strategies offer some steps towards what otherwise might seem an impossible journey.

Epilogue

I started this journey wanting to give voice to experiences of bullying and toxicity in the health professions. Others will be the judge of how successful or otherwise I have been. I believed understanding what happened to others would help me make sense of my own experiences. I didn't realise how much. I have so much compassion for the champions. What they went through and how this changed the course of their careers and lives has helped me do something I find challenging, to have compassion for myself. I might not be quite there yet, but I feel less guilty thinking others had it so much worse than me. No amount of bullying can be justified. I have forgiven myself for the fact that I couldn't make the bullying stop, that I said or did the wrong things, or didn't say or do the right things. I'd love to say the ruminations have stopped. At least, they are much less frequent. I have learned to accept what happened without justifying it or taking the blame.

The champions have taken me on a journey towards recognising bullying as trauma. Bullying is a form of abuse. It causes distress, often severe distress. It is not something we simply need to "get over". We don't need to become "more resilient" and learn to deal with a toxic workplace. We don't need to be told we should "just leave" if we are unhappy or that we should "stand up" to the bully and refuse to allow it to happen. These glib platitudes don't "get" the impact of bullying, and the powerlessness targets often feel. They do not acknowledge that we have suffered mistreatment and abuse and need to be heard and supported. There is no magic wand to wave to make bullying go away, and it will never go away when people's stories are not listened to and accepted as real for them.

People who have been bullied need to grieve. They need to process the loss of the job they loved the same way they would grieve the loss of a limb. Surely the words of the champions have shown so clearly how profoundly their lives have changed. Wanting to move on does not make it happen. Being told to move on does not make it happen. We need to grieve in our own way, in our own timeframe.

I conclude this book by sharing some updates from the champions since our last conversations:

Sam recently decided enough was enough and formally met with a senior manager to put her bullying experiences "on the table". She is still apprehensive about potential consequences but feels supported in considering her options.

B. Happell, *Sickness in Health: Bullying in Nursing and other Health Professions*, https://doi.org/10.1007/978-3-031-49336-2

Terry has secured a long-term job that will enable him to stay in Australia and start living the dream he came here for.

Rory successfully completed the requirements to become a Fellow of her Specialist College.

Alex finally settled the case with the Ambulance Service. She is now looking at moving on with her life without their continual presence in the background.

My sincere gratitude to you, the champions. I can't thank you enough for making this book a reality and teaching me so much. I hope it has also been valuable for you. Some of you thanked me for the opportunity to talk about these experiences. You said it helped even just a little on the healing journey. Your support of and belief in this book kept me going when I doubted it could become a reality. You truly are champions.

After reading the book, some champions made comments. I found them touching and compelling. With their permission, I am including them here.

Shannon: I learnt so much from the book. I have applied that to my working life! I thoroughly enjoyed reading it. It gave me great insight into others' behaviours and my enabling behaviours that may allow others to get away with it! After reading the book, I developed such insight into the different forms of bullying, and I can apply my knowledge across the lifespan. I have a primary school-aged son to a 23-year-old daughter who also works in healthcare, and she has had her share of bullying in the workplace. She loved it and now can identify early warning signs!

Alex: You've done a beautiful job not just for me but all the other people who have been traumatised. It's hard to read, but at the same time, it gives us all something that feels stripped from us, our humanity and voice. I've felt for 5 years that the employer I am still tied to, who has complete control over my health and life, doesn't even consider me a human. Thank you for recognising and highlighting the humanity in all of us. I'm so grateful, thank you.

Taylor: This is such an important and great book! You should feel so proud of what you have achieved here and what this book will achieve. What a powerful legacy you are leaving in this book!

Chris: Amazing. Loved the way you made sense of all our stories. It does a great job of providing insight into different types of bullying behaviours and the very real human impacts of being on the receiving end of these.

Sam: In a strange way, it's affirming, reading not only my story but the others. Affirming, knowing it's not okay.

I am realistic. This book is not a magic wand to end bullying. I hope it contributes to conversations and helps to change our understanding of what bullying is. If the book provides comfort to even one person, encourages them to think differently about bullying, see the need for change, and recognise toxic behaviour as not okay, this has all been worth it.